USING YOUR HEAD TO LAND ON YOUR FEET: A BEGINNING NURSE'S GUIDE TO CRITICAL THINKING

Stephen Brookfield's Four Critical Thinking Processes

The questions that follow each of the four major critical thinking processes will help you focus your thinking about the immediate situation.

CONTEXTUAL AWARENESS AND DECIDING WHAT TO OBSERVE AND CONSIDER

This includes an awareness of what's happening in the context of the situation, including values, cultural issues, and environmental influences. Sample questions include:

- What was going on in the situation that may have influenced the outcome?
- What factors influenced my behavior and others' behavior in this situation?
- What else was happening simultaneously that affected me in this situation?
- What happened just before this incident that made a difference?
- What emotional responses influenced how I was reacting in this situation?

- What else do I need to know? What information is missing?
- How do I go about getting the information I need?
- What about this situation have I seen before? What is different/dissimilar?
- Who should have been involved in order to improve the outcome?
- What's important and what's not important in this situation?
- What changes in behavior alerted me that something was wrong?

EXPLORING AND IMAGINING ALTERNATIVES

This involves exploring as many alternatives as you can think of for the given situation. Sample questions include:

- What is one possible explanation for [insert what is happening?]
- What are other explanations for what is happening?
- What is one thing I could do in this situation?
- What are two more possibilities/other alternatives?
- What else would I want to know in this situation?

- Are there others who might be able to help me develop more alternatives?
- Of the possible actions I am considering, which one is most reasonable? Why are the others not as reasonable?
- Are there other resources that need to be mobilized?

USING YOUR HEAD TO LAND ON YOUR FEET: A BEGINNING NURSE'S GUIDE TO CRITICAL THINKING

Bonnie Raingruber, RN, PhD
Professor of Nursing
and

Ann Haffer, RN, EdD
Professor of Nursing

College of Health and Human Services
Division of Nursing
California State University
Sacramento, California

F. A. DAVIS COMPANY / PUBLISHERS • PHILADELPHIA

F. A. Davis Company
1915 Arch Street
Philadelphia, PA 19103
www.fadavis.com

Printed in the United States of America

Last digit indicates print number: 10 9 8 7 6 5

Acquisitions Editor: Melanie Freely
Developmental Editor: Marilyn Kochman
Production Editor: Jessica Howie Martin
Cover Designer: Louis J. Forgione

As new scientific information becomes available through basic and clinical research, recommended treatments and drug therapies undergo changes. The authors and publisher have done everything possible to make this book accurate, up to date, and in accord with accepted standards at the time of publication. The authors, editors, and publisher are not responsible for errors or omissions or for consequences from application of the book, and make no warranty, expressed or implied, in regard to the contents of the book. Any practice described in this book should be applied by the reader in accordance with professional standards of care used in regard to the unique circumstances that may apply in each situation. The reader is advised always to check product information (package inserts) for changes and new information regarding dose and contraindications before administering any drug. Caution is especially urged when using new or infrequently ordered drugs.

Library of Congress Cataloging-in-Publication Data

Raingruber, Bonnie.
   Using your head to land on your feet : a beginning nurse's guide to critical thinking / Bonnie Raingruber, Ann Haffer.
     p. cm.
   Includes bibliographical references and index.
   ISBN 10: 0-8036-0606-0 (pbk.)   ISBN 13: 978-0-8036-0606-7 (pbk.)
    1. Nursing—Examinations, questions, etc. 2. Critical thinking—Examinations, questions, etc. I. Haffer, Ann. II. Title.
RT 86.R35 2001
610.73′076—dc21

2001017285

This book is dedicated to Dr. Patricia Benner in recognition of her pioneering work in skill progression, clinical reasoning, ethical decision making, and caring practices within nursing. Her work helped shape the development and structure of the clinical reasoning and critical thinking course at California State University, Sacramento, from which this book derived. Patricia Benner embodies what is meant by the words scholar, mentor, and educator.

PREFACE

Most beginners agree that clinical experiences are the most anxiety-producing events of their careers. Nurses help patients survive life-threatening situations every day, and when beginners finally put their skills and knowledge to the test in real-life situations, it can be overwhelming indeed. They soon learn that classroom knowledge is not enough to succeed on the job. They also need experience, confidence, and—most important—the ability to think critically and exercise sound reasoning skills. These are the strengths that enable nurses to respond to unexpected situations, prioritize responsibilities, advocate for their patients, and, despite continual pressure and conflicting demands, provide patients with the best health care possible.

In today's rapidly changing health-care environment, it is more important than ever for nurses to be prepared for clinical challenges. Patient acuities are consistently high and patients are hospitalized for shorter periods of time. Additionally, staff-patient ratios are decreasing, and nurses often float to other units in the hospital, assuming greater responsibility for a broader spectrum of patient assignments. Yet beginners lack the experience necessary for operating most effectively in this environment.

Using Your Head To Land On Your Feet: A Beginning Nurse's Guide To Critical Thinking was designed to add to your experience. This interactive text includes more than 50 narratives related by senior students and beginning nurses who have taken our Reasoning courses at California State University, Sacramento. The narratives, presented in authentic dialogue, highlight the reasoning problems encountered when students begin clinical and describe situations in medical-surgical, maternal-child, community health, and mental health nursing. Our students report that when they hear other beginners' stories, they are reassured that they are on target in their skill level development. Students also say that hearing others' clinical stories is like being in the situation; the stories become part of their clinical reasoning memory.

Unlike case studies, which provide only pertinent details, narratives include descriptions of contextual factors beyond the immediate focus, providing the complexities actually seen in clinical practice. They provide excellent learning opportunities because there is more than one right answer, and beginners are challenged to consider many aspects of a situation. Critical thinking is not discussed in theory; it is applied to accounts of real-life situations that represent stumbling blocks in beginners' reasoning abilities.

After each scenario we present questions, derived from the four critical thinking processes suggested by Stephen Brookfield, known for his ideas about critical thinking and reflective practices, particularly as they relate to adult learning. We have indicated, in italics, which thinking process the question is derived from. The questions help focus attention on the chapter's reasoning problems, foster habits of reflection, and identify relevant decision points and assessment findings. Questions frequently ask you to compare your experiences and responses to those presented in the scenario. This helps you decide what to do in similar future situations. The questions also highlight how emotion and being involved with the patient can affect the development of reasoning skill.

In addition to Brookfield's questions, we have included others related to the specific clinical reasoning problem represented in the chapter. These questions are designated as (*Chapter reasoning problem*).

In each chapter we have also included narratives presented by experienced nurses so you can see the differences in thought processes and behaviors between experienced and beginning nurses.

Mind Maps

In addition to real-life scenarios and reasoning questions, the text introduces you to mind maps. These are visual tools that help you identify important elements in a situation and understand their relationship with one another. Chapter 1 describes mind maps in more detail.

Chapter Content

Each chapter focuses on one of the significant reasoning problems or blocks that beginners commonly experience. However, in actual practice, all of these problems are interrelated and rarely occur in isolation.

Chapter 1 introduces you to Brookfield's questions and the concept of mind mapping. Chapter 2 describes problems that can occur when you encounter unexpected events that interrupt established routines. Beginners report that they become frozen in their tracks, unable to think or make decisions, and that they remain scattered and disorganized for long periods. The questioning approaches in the chapter help students and beginners identify ways in which they can mobilize their thinking and their ability to act.

Chapter 3 addresses the questioning processes involved in critical thinking and reasoning. Students and beginners say they are uncomfortable asking questions. They feel they cannot doubt or challenge the judgments or actions of more experienced professionals. Beginners also feel they should already know the answers to most of their questions, that they will look "dumb" or irritate more experienced practitioners. In spite of their reluctance, they nonetheless ask numerous questions. This chapter helps beginners gain confidence in seeking information and in asserting themselves when they question others' responses.

Chapter 4 discusses the need to stay open to possibilities. Beginners tend to consider only one or two, and then act on those rather than continuing to look for other options until all the pieces fit (Benner, Tanner & Chesla, 1996). The narratives in this chapter highlight the need to stay open until you feel assured you have explored all reasonable options; the stories also illustrate why it is important to anticipate future possibilities.

When beginners confront ethical dilemmas, they often have difficulty knowing how to advocate for their patients. Chapter 5 focuses on ethical decision making, ways of connecting with patients, and suggestions for developing advocacy skills.

This book is designed for nursing students to use throughout their program once they have completed their introductory clinical course work. It will also be useful for nurses who are just beginning their clinical practice. Until nurses have acquired a substantial amount of experience, their reasoning is not yet highly developed and they may continue to experience reasoning blocks like those described in the chapters.

Throughout the book we use the term "beginner" to mean either a student or a beginning nurse. We think there is little or no difference in the clinical reasoning of advanced students and nurses with fewer than 2 years of experience (Benner, Tanner & Chesla, 1996). The experienced nurses whose scenarios appear in this book had been in clinical practice for 4 or more years when they described their scenarios.

How To Use This Book

You may use this book either individually or in a group setting. If you work alone, you should complete this workbook as a self-paced module. Collaborative group-learning approaches, in which scenarios are discussed and questions answered, can be especially helpful. When beginners hear their peers' thoughts and responses to specific narratives, it confirms their reasoning.

Some instructors may use certain narratives as part of a classroom discussion to complement study in particular clinical areas. Other narratives might be assigned as homework.

We recommend that you answer workbook questions in short sentences or phrases that capture significant concepts. Also keep in mind that there may be more than one correct response to many of the questions, as is the case in actual clinical practice.

You may progress through the chapters in any order, but be sure to read all of the scenarios in each. Remember, repetitive experiences are crucial for facilitating skill development and building reflective habits.

BONNIE RAINGRUBER
ANN HAFFER

CONSULTANTS AND REVIEWERS

Barbara Matthews Blanton, BSN, MSN
Clinical Instructor
Texas Woman's University
Denton, Texas

Linda Kelly Brown, BSN, MA
Professor
New Hampshire Community Technical
    College
Claremont, New Hampshire

Joseph Catalano, BSN, MSN, PhD
Professor
East Central University
Ada, Oklahoma

Terry DeVito, RN, MEd
Coordinator/Assistant Professor
Capital Community Technical College
Hartford, Connecticut

Emily Drosk-Bielak, BSN, MS, PhD
Associate Professor
Grand Valley State University
Allendale, Michigan

Claretta Dupree, RN, MSN, PhD
Associate Professor
North Park University
Chicago, Illinois

Kelly Fisher, RN, MS
Assistant Professor
Simmons College
Boston, Massachusetts

Joan Fleitas, EdD
Associate Professor of Nursing
Fairfield University
Fairfield, Connecticut

Alicia M. Horkan, MSN
Assistant Professor
Simmons College
Boston, Massachusetts

Susan J. W. Hsia, RN, PhD
Associate Professor
Washburn University
Topeka, Kansas

Lynne Kreutzer-Baraglia, MS
Administrative Dean
Concordia University and West Suburban
    College of Nursing
Oak Park, Illinois

Barbara Murray, BS, MS
Associate Professor
University of Vermont
Burlington, Vermont

Jane Rapps, DNSc
Associate Professor
San Diego State University
San Diego, California

Deborah Roush, MSN
Assistant Professor
Valdosta State University
Valdosta, Georgia

Pam Schuster, RN, PhD
Associate Professor
Youngstown State University
Department of Nursing
Youngstown, Ohio

Susan R. Seager, RN, MSN, EdD
Associate Professor
Middle Tennessee State University
Murfreesboro, Tennessee

Elizabeth Shannon, BSN, MSN, CPNP
Assistant Professor
Simmons College
Boston, Massachusetts

Marilyn Smith-Stoner
Adjunct Faculty
University of Phoenix
Phoenix, Arizona

Peggy Trueman, RN, BS, BSN, MSN, CS
Instructor
Gaston College
Dallas, North Carolina

Pat Woodbury, BSN, MSN, ARNP-C
Professor
Valencia Community College
Orlando, Florida

CONTENTS

CHAPTER **1**

APPROACHES FOR DEVELOPING CRITICAL
THINKING HABITS   1

CHAPTER **2**

WHAT TO DO WHEN YOU DON'T KNOW
WHAT TO DO
SCATTERED? DISORGANIZED? FROZEN?   11

CHAPTER **3**

THE POWER OF QUESTIONING   55

CHAPTER **4**

STAYING OPEN TO POSSIBILITIES
LEARNING TO ASK "WHAT ELSE?" AND
"WHAT IF?"   95

CHAPTER **5**

THE ART OF MAKING ETHICAL DECISIONS   137

REFERENCES   183

INDEX   185

APPROACHES FOR DEVELOPING CRITICAL THINKING HABITS

Sound Familiar?

- ☐ I tend to follow a similar routine every day.

- ☐ So many things need to be done, I have trouble deciding what to do first.

- ☐ I focus on tasks that need to be completed.

- ☐ When I see something that is not right in a patient, I usually ask for help from a more experienced nurse.

- ☐ When something unexpected occurs, or interferes with routines, I have difficulty thinking and making decisions. I freeze in my tracks.

- ☐ Sometimes I view patients through blinders. I realize later that there were things I should have noticed, but never saw.

- ☐ After something unusual happens, I remain disorganized for quite a while.

- ☐ I often stop asking questions before I feel sure of the answer I'm getting.

- ☐ I sometimes feel I should be more assertive about asking questions, instead of allowing others to influence my actions.

- ☐ When I see a change in a patient's condition, I tend to focus on only one or two possible explanations or causes for the change.

- ☐ I tend to rely on my first impression instead of considering other options.

- ☐ I take copious notes to help me remember things and stay organized.

- ☐ I use other nurses' charting as a guide for my own.

- ☐ The potential for harming my patients is frightening to me.

- ☐ I don't always know how to advocate for my patients.

Do any of these behaviors and reactions sound familiar? If you are a beginner, we suspect you will answer "yes." These behaviors and reactions reflect the beginner's lack of practical, real-world clinical experience necessary to guide thinking and actions. Beginners have a limited supply of past clinical experiences to serve as guides for their thinking and actions. Collecting experiences and reflecting on them so they can be easily retrieved when similar experiences occur in the future will help beginners progress (*Benner, Tanner & Chesla, 1996*).

OBJECTIVES
After completing the learning experiences in this chapter, you will be able to:

- Analyze and learn from your and others' clinical experience by writing and listening to narrative accounts.
- Learn how to apply Stephen Brookfield's critical thinking processes.

- Develop mind maps to help you visualize ways to solve problems.
- Recognize the value of keeping a reflective journal that can help you grow professionally.

A Short Scenario

Here is an example of a clinical story that was so vivid in this nurse's memory that it later changed her practice.

Sally got report from the night nurse, who suggested her patients were mostly stable except for one diabetic patient whose blood sugars had been very labile. Sally had taken the night nurse's report without question and began assessing her patients, starting with the most acute patient and progressing to the least acute. But when she reached the last room and opened the door, she heard breathing that sounded like a washing machine.

Sally could see that the patient, Ruth, was in trouble: she was sitting bolt upright, using her whole body to breathe. Sally was surprised because Ruth, who was in end-stage renal failure, had been dialyzed the day before. Sally's first thought was, "I need to suction this patient fast!" But there was no suction setup in the room, so Sally asked the ward clerk to quickly get the equipment. When Sally finally started suctioning Ruth, it didn't help.

Sally then decided Ruth needed dialysis to remove some of the fluid, and arranged to get this started. But before dialysis could work, Ruth started to arrest and was coded. She had been alert and oriented until shortly before the code was called. Ruth grabbed Sally's stethoscope, pulled her close to her face and gasped, "I'm dying, aren't I?" Because Sally knew Ruth well from many previous admissions, Sally answered honestly that it was possible Ruth was dying. Unfortunately, the code was unsuccessful and Ruth died.

Sally tearfully ended her story saying that after that experience, she learned to always do a quick check of all her patients at the beginning of the shift rather than assessing each one, based on acuities from the morning report.

Have you ever talked to a friend or colleague about a frightening or surprising incident, like Sally's, that happened during your clinical experiences? Have others ever done the same with you? Can you think of a clinical story someone told you that you never forgot and that influenced the way you practice?

Throughout their careers nurses share stories and talk to each other about issues that concern them in their clinical practice. This communication exchange helps nurses learn, builds confidence, and passes on common traditions and practices (*Kirkpatrick, Ford & Castelloe, 1997*). When placed in a formal context and accompanied by guided reflection and questions, these stories provide powerful opportunities to improve critical thinking skills.

What is critical thinking? Although widely regarded as a component of clinical reasoning and decision making, critical thinking is difficult to define. It is a multifaceted process that includes logical, rhetorical, and humanistic skills and attitudes that promote the ability to determine what one should believe and do. Critical thinking requires one to actively process and evaluate information, to validate existing knowledge, and to create new knowledge. It involves reflective thinking.

Four Critical Thinking Approaches

In this chapter, we introduce four approaches to help you develop habits of reflection and critical thinking skills. The first approach (Critical Thinking Approach #1) is reading and reflecting on narratives like the opening story to add to your repertoire of clinical experiences. The second is answering a series of questions derived from the four critical thinking processes suggested by Stephen Brookfield. The third is creating mind maps to help you identify ways to deal with reasoning problems. The fourth is keeping a journal to help you develop reflective habits.

Critical Thinking Approach #2: Stephen Brookfield's Four Critical Thinking Processes

The questions that follow each of the following four major critical thinking processes will help you focus your thinking about the immediate situation.

CONTEXTUAL AWARENESS AND DECIDING WHAT TO OBSERVE AND CONSIDER

This includes an awareness of what's happening in the context of the situation, including values, cultural issues, and environmental influences. Sample questions include:

- What was going on in this situation that may have influenced the outcome?
- What factors influenced my behavior and others' behavior in this situation?
- What else was happening simultaneously that affected me in this situation?
- What happened just before this incident occurred that made a difference?
- What emotional responses influenced how I was reacting in this situation?
- What else do I need to know? What information is missing?
- How do I go about getting the information I need?
- What about this situation have I seen before? What is different/dissimilar?
- Who should have been involved in order to improve the outcome?
- What's important and what's not important in this situation?
- What changes in behavior alerted me that something was wrong?

EXPLORING AND IMAGINING ALTERNATIVES

This involves thinking about and imagining other ways of looking at the situation, not just the first thing that comes to your mind. It involves exploring as many alternatives as you can think of for the given situation. Sample questions include:

- What is one possible explanation for [insert what is happening]?
- What are other explanations for what is happening?
- What is one thing I could do in this situation?
- What are two more possibilities/other alternatives?
- What else would I want to know in this situation?
- Are there others who might be able to help me develop more alternatives?

- Of the possible actions I am considering, which one is most reasonable? Why are the others not as reasonable?
- Are there other resources that need to be mobilized?

ASSUMPTION RECOGNITION AND ANALYSIS

This involves analyzing assumptions you are making about the situation as well as examining the beliefs that underlie your choices. Sample questions include:

- What has been taken for granted in this situation?
- Which beliefs/values shaped my assumptions?
- What assumptions contributed to the problem in this situation?
- What rationale supports my assumptions?
- How will I know my assumption is correct?

REFLECTIVE SKEPTICISM/DECIDING WHAT TO DO

This critical thinking approach involves questioning, analyzing, and reflecting on the rationale for decisions. Sample questions include:

- Am I sure of my interpretation in this situation?
- What rationale do I have for my decisions?
- What aspects of this situation require the most careful attention?
- Why was it important to intervene?
- What got me started taking some action?
- In priority order, identify what I would do in this situation and why.
- What priorities were missed?
- Having decided what was wrong/happening, what is the best response?
- What might I delegate in this situation?
- What was done? Why was it done?
- What would I do differently in the future, after reflecting on this situation?
- What else might work in this situation?

Let's use Sally's scenario to demonstrate how the Brookfield-derived questions can help you develop your critical thinking skills by applying them to accounts of real-life situations. [Please note: It is not necessary to consider each question for every clinical situation. Reflect on only those questions that apply to the particular situation, but be sure to consider at least some of the questions in each category, as illustrated below.]

CONTEXTUAL AWARENESS AND DECIDING WHAT TO OBSERVE AND CONSIDER

- What major factors influenced Sally's behavior?

The night nurse had suggested that the patients were mostly stable, and Sally took the report without question. There was no suction setup in the room, which delayed respiratory intervention. Sally knew Ruth from previous admissions, and her response was based on her knowledge of the patient's usual clinical course after dialysis. Ruth's apparent need for an honest answer influenced Sally's comment to Ruth that she could be dying.

- What else did Sally need to know? What information was missing?

Sally needed a more detailed report. The night nurse's assessment of how Ruth was doing was not accurate. It would have helped if Sally had more information about Ruth's lung sounds, her creatinine level (to assess the degree of her renal failure), and the reason she had not called for the nurse earlier using her call bell.

EXPLORING AND IMAGINING ALTERNATIVES

● What is one thing Sally could have done differently in this situation?

She could have begun the shift by quickly assessing all the patients, rather than relying on the night nurse's assessment acuities.

● What else could Sally have done?

She could have called the code team as soon as she heard the breath sounds and saw the patient's distress; she could have checked the room for equipment.

ASSUMPTION RECOGNITION AND ANALYSIS

● What did Sally take for granted in this situation?

Sally assumed the night nurse's report was accurate; that Ruth had been dialyzed the day before and would be stable for a while; that suctioning would make a difference at this point; that Ruth wanted to know the truth; and that she had a good relationship with Ruth.

● Which beliefs/values shaped Sally's assumptions?

Sally was honest because she knew Ruth pretty well and knew Ruth was dying.

REFLECTIVE SKEPTICISM/DECIDING WHAT TO DO

● What was Sally's rationale for her decisions?

The night nurse had said the patients were mostly stable except for one diabetic patient, so Sally assessed by acuity and visited the diabetic patient first. In the past, Ruth had done very well after dialysis, so Sally assumed Ruth would be stable because her fluids had been managed by the previous day's dialysis. Sally suctioned, rather than waiting for dialysis, because the effects would be immediate.

● What made Sally start taking some action?

When Sally opened the door, she noticed that Ruth's breathing sounded like a washing machine. Ruth was obviously in severe respiratory distress, using her whole body to breathe.

Critical Thinking Approach #3: Mind Maps

A mind map is a visual learning tool that will help you identify key elements in a situation and understand their relationship with one another. It is based on the assumption that association plays a major role in nearly every mental function, including problem solving. Mind maps graphically depict associated thoughts

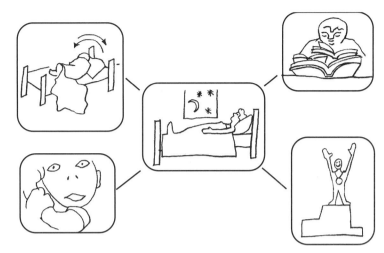

FIGURE 1-1 Picture mind map. The night before your first day of clinical can be anxiety provoking. To avoid a restless night, you may consider reviewing a text, visualizing success, or calling a friend for support.

and ideas, help you discover what might not have been clear before, and help you generate solutions to problems. In a sense, a mind map is a visual record of your thoughts.

To begin a mind map, you draw a word or picture in the center of a piece of paper to represent the main focus of the map. As ideas emerge, you place words or pictures around the main idea to illustrate how they relate to each other and to the central theme.

The following example illustrates how mind maps work. The central theme of the mind map is "The Night Before." For students about to begin clinical experiences, or nurses starting a new job or floating to a different unit, these experiences may evoke anxiety as well as ideas on how to cope with the anxiety.

To create the mind map, place "The Night Before" in the center of the page and arrange the associated thoughts (toss and turn, call friends, review books, visualize success) around the main theme. You may use pictures, words, or a combination of both to create your mind map. Figure 1-1 is an example of a picture mind map.

Do any of these behaviors look familiar? When you have felt anxious about events that would be occurring the next day, have you ever called someone to gain support or information? Maybe you turned to nursing texts or pharmacology books to refresh your memory. Perhaps you had a wakeful night, or tossed and turned all night. Maybe you thought about past successes because doing this helped you calm your fears. Can you think of any other pictures that would apply to this situation?

Some people prefer thinking in words rather than in pictures. Below is a version of the same mind map using words instead of pictures (Fig 1-2).

In each of the next four chapters, we ask you to develop a mind map based on the reasoning problems presented in the scenarios. Like the previous examples, your mind map should show both the problems and the ways of dealing with them. When something happens in the future that is similar to the stories in the narratives, you should be able to recall the solutions and coping approaches depicted in your mind maps.

In clinical practice, you should develop a mind map after a problematic situation has occurred. Physically arranging records of your thoughts and ideas on a

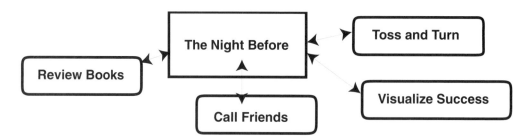

FIGURE 1-2 Word mind map.

piece of paper will help you improve your responses to a similar situation in the future.

Critical Thinking Approach #4: Journal

We also recommend that you begin to keep a journal of clinical experiences that were troubling to you. Think about what bothered you and what you would do differently in the future. This form of reflecting on a consistent basis will enhance your developing reasoning skills. Reflection allows you to view your own thinking, reasoning, and actions. It helps you create and clarify meaning and new understandings of a particular experience. It involves putting events into a perspective that is more easily recalled. When you again encounter a similar situation, you should be able to recall what you did (or what you would do differently) as well as the reasoning behind your actions. If enough similar events occur in your experiences, your reasoning and actions can become almost second nature. When this happens, dealing with clinical situations is easier.

tips!   Keep a reflective journal.

REFLECTIVE JOURNAL

CHAPTER 2

WHAT TO DO WHEN YOU DON'T KNOW WHAT TO DO

SCATTERED? DISORGANIZED? FROZEN?

Sound Familiar?

○ I feel scattered and lose my focus. It seems like I am out of control.

○ I get overwhelmed and do pointless things. I go around in circles and can't think what to do first.

○ My mind can suddenly go blank and I can't think what to do.

○ I freeze and don't do anything at all.

○ I have to stop to think about what to do next.

○ I get off track and stay disorganized for what seems to be a long time.

When something unexpected happens or your usual routines are interrupted, which of the above behaviors describe you?

OBJECTIVES

After completing the learning experiences in this chapter, you will be able to:

● Recognize the influence of routines in your nursing approaches.

● Identify situations that lead to freezing and feeling very disorganized.

● Become aware of your freezing responses.

● Develop strategies for moving beyond being scattered and/or disorganized in clinical settings.

A Short Scenario

Help! My Mind Just Went Blank

Imagine yourself in an acute-care clinical situation. You have gotten report and have started your morning routines. Everything is going as planned. It's about 7:45 AM, and you are about to start preparing your medications. Suddenly a patient's daughter rushes toward you and says, "My father, Mr. Peary, in room 209, is spitting up blood." He looked fine a few minutes ago. You walk rapidly toward the patient's room, thinking, "Help! What am I going to do when I get to the room? I have to get the oxygen humidifier for the patient in 202. His nose was burning him and his wife is waiting for me to come right back. What could be happening with Mr. Peary?"

You enter the room, and the first thing you think is: "He's lying flat." You say to yourself, "Better elevate his head. That's what I did up on the respiratory unit where I recently worked for 2 months." The daughter tells you the patient spat some blood into the emesis basin. You ask to see the basin, and sure enough, there is a small amount of bright red blood in it. You don't know what to do next. Another RN stops by and says the wife of the patient in 202 is asking about the burning in her husband's nose again. Your mind doesn't seem to be able to think about anything. The nurse says she will take over with Mr. Peary while you follow up with the patient in room 202. Later you recall the situation and can't believe you didn't take Mr. Peary's blood pressure, count respirations, ask about pain, or listen to his lungs or anything else. You just raised his head. You wonder why you missed so many things.

Have you ever experienced anything like this? What happened to your ability to stay focused and organized after this or some comparable unexpected situation occurred? Were you able to take immediate, reasoned action?

In clinical situations, beginning nurses and students tend to focus primarily on their routines (*Benner, Tanner, & Chesla, 1996; Haffer, 1990*). Their goal is to get a list of tasks done like ordered treatments, assessments, routine care, and charting. When something interrupts these routines, beginners become disorganized, sometimes for the rest of the shift.

Beginners have described a variety of situations in which "freezing" occurred in response to a clinical situation they perceived to be a crisis. Something unexpected happened, and the beginners reported their mind suddenly went blank. They felt like they were paralyzed and could not remember what to do next. Others described a sense of being overwhelmed, a dithering back and forth doing pointless things and feeling scattered. They perceived things were happening to them and they felt out of control. They reported acting in a rote manner, doing routine activities that were not appropriately prioritized. It could be said their abilities to reason, plan, and take action became stalled or frozen.

Recall a Scenario

Recall a time in your clinical practice when your mind went blank, when you couldn't think what to do next, or you more or less froze in response to an unexpected situation. Describe what happened in as much detail as possible. Think of the description as a painting or a picture. Pretend you're telling a story in which you include details like your Great-Aunt Mildred did when she went on and on. Describe what you saw, heard, felt, and looked for as you made decisions. Also include hunches you derived and ruled out, and explain why.

Be sure to include environmental factors, such as the time of day, people involved, temperaments, moods, and your concerns. In other words, describe anything you did or said. This will help you examine the relevant critical thinking and clinical reasoning problems discussed in the chapter as well as ways to deal with them.

Write Your Scenario Here

After you write your scenario, answer the questions below. They are designed to help you develop your reasoning skills and find ways to deal with or manage the stumbling blocks to your reasoning. At least one question is included from each of Stephen Brookfield's four critical thinking processes, and at least one focuses on the reasoning problem or stumbling block presented in the chapter. As a reminder, the Brookfield process from which each question is derived will be in italic, and the questions pertaining to the chapter's reasoning problem will be followed by (*Chapter reasoning problem*).

THINKING IT THROUGH

1. What was going on in the situation that influenced what was happening and caused you to lose your ability to think and plan what to do next? (*Contextual awareness and deciding what to observe and consider*)

2. Are there others who might have helped you to develop more alternatives? What would your peers, instructor, or nursing preceptor suggest you might have done? (*Exploring and imagining alternatives*)

3. Were you able to back up your assumptions with rationale? (*Assumption recognition and analysis*)

4. What would you do differently in this situation after having a chance to reflect on it? (*Reflective skepticism/deciding what to do*)

5. Describe what happened to trigger your freezing episode and what helped to get you back on track in your clinical practice in this scenario. (*Chapter reasoning problem*) (Fig. 2-1)

Freezing Scenarios

Each of the following scenarios is followed by several questions to help you reflect about what has occurred. The questions should help you understand your own approaches to overcoming your tendency to freeze. Be sure to pay attention

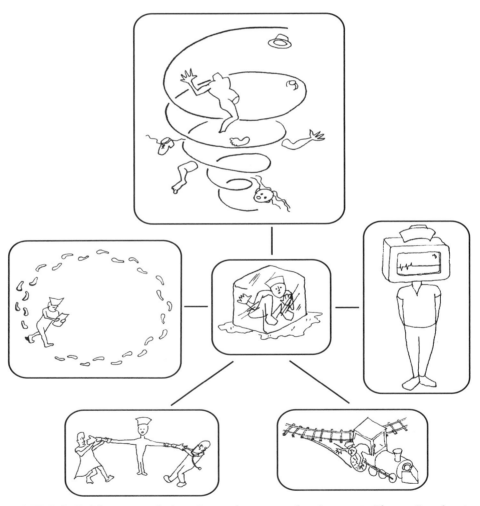

FIGURE 2-1 Unexpected situations often cause beginners to "freeze" and not know what to do next. They may feel they're being pulled apart, their minds are going blank, they're being pulled in two different directions, getting off track, or going around in circles.

to the recurring problems you see and to formulate alternate approaches. At the end of the chapter you will develop your own mind map about your insights and coping approaches.

Why Didn't I Think to Ask That?

I was caring for three patients and was expecting a fourth at any time. Things were pretty hectic on the unit and in the hospital that day, but I seemed to be managing my patient load well. As soon as one patient was discharged, another arrived on the unit. There was little idle conversation between the nurses; instead there were just brief exchanges at the med cart. I got a call from the recovery room nurse, who was anxious to give report and transfer the patient. The patient was a 43-year-old female with a previous neck resection related to laryngeal cancer. She was readmitted for dysphasia and a substantial weight loss. A jejunostomy was performed so that parenteral feeds could take place. The report I got was really brief; it said the procedure had been tolerated well and vital signs were within normal limits. I thought this was going to be a "cakewalk," so I informed my preceptor of the patient's status and volunteered to do the admission assessment.

When the patient arrived, I was completing a wet-to-dry dressing change on another patient and was not able to assist in the bed transfer. When I did get into her room, the new patient was requesting a pen and paper. She wrote, "I need more air." She was getting oxygen. The recovery room nurse had assessed her lungs, charted that she sounded a little congested, and did nothing further. I listened to her lungs and she did sound congested. I thought maybe she needed to be suctioned, but the room was not set up for suctioning. I ran to the utility room to gather the equipment, but my mind went blank and I could not remember all the parts I needed. I told another floor nurse, and she helped me.

We took the vitals, which were: temperature = 38.2, pulse = 84, respiratory rate = 22, and blood pressure = 184/100. The recovery room nurse had failed to mention that the patient had a history of hypertension. Fortunately, the nurse who was helping me had cared for this patient before and knew her history. She told me to contact the house officer for nifedipine. The med was ordered and I gave it. When I got back into the room her blood pressure was 92/52.

My preceptor told me that I should have monitored the patient every 5 minutes until I was sure she had stabilized. Her blood pressure did creep up to 118/68 and my crisis ended, but I was pretty shaken afterwards because I had taken so many things for granted. I never should have accepted such a short report. I should have asked for specific measurements and a brief patient history. The patient should not have gone into the room until I had checked it and made sure it was set up appropriately. I did not have a clue about the former neck resection surgery and the possibility of the patient's having a permanent trach. I froze. I administered a med to a patient and did not observe her for possible complications afterward. I should have prioritized what I was doing. The dressing change could have waited. This situation helped me learn to take nothing for granted and to be prepared for the unexpected.

THINKING IT THROUGH

Below are questions to guide your thinking about the above scenario. Because this is the first one, we have included answers as examples of appropriate responses. Please remember that there may be others that are also correct. The important thing is for you to think about the scenario and to generate your own responses. (Expert nurses would typically answer these questions in much greater detail because they would be able to generate more possibilities than a beginner's experience would allow. We have modeled sample answers corresponding closely to a beginner's level of reasoning skill.)

1. What was going on in the situation that influenced what was happening? (*Contextual awareness and deciding what to observe and consider*)

    ● Nurses were hurried, distracted.
    ● The recovery room nurse was in a hurry.
    ● The beginner had limited knowledge of patient's history.
    ● She was interrupted while doing a dressing change when the patient arrived.
    ● She did not admit the patient herself, had not checked the room, was not aware of missing suction.

2. What information was missing in this situation? What else would you have wanted to know when you admitted this patient? (*Contextual awareness and deciding what to observe and consider*)

    ● Patient's history
    ● Extent of cancer
    ● Permanent tracheostomy
    ● Pre-op vital signs and use of oxygen
    ● Time nifedipine was given and patient's individual response to this medication
    ● Extent/length/events of surgery
    ● Recovery room course—including vital signs
    ● How long after surgery the temperature began to elevate

3. What about this situation is similar to something you have seen before and what is different? (*Contextual awareness and deciding what to observe and consider*)

    ● Have received patients after getting short, sketchy reports when I was busy and very distracted. They were always more acute than anticipated. I have never taken care of a jejunostomy patient immediately postop.

4. What was one possible explanation for why this patient's blood pressure dropped? (*Exploring and imagining alternatives*)

    ● Events of surgery and PACU (post-anesthesia care unit)
    ● Response to nifedipine
    ● Transferring from PACU cart to bed (if blood pressure drop occurred immediately after)

5. The beginner in this scenario identified several alternative courses of action she wished she had completed. What were they? (*Exploring and imagining alternatives*)

- Determined the patient's history
- Taken vital signs to monitor for medication effects
- Checked the room setup before admission
- Waited to do the dressing change
- Gotten a more complete report from the recovery room nurse

6. This beginner reasoned that the patient's "need for more air" was caused by a need for suctioning. Would you have made the same decision? What other possible explanations are there for what happened? (*Exploring and imagining alternatives*)

- May have made the same decision about suctioning. Would have depended on chest and breath sounds.
- Anxiety, congestive heart failure, hypotension.

7. What was taken for granted in this situation? How would you know this assumption is correct/incorrect? (*Assumption recognition and analysis*)

- Taking care of this patient would be simple—incorrect, as evidenced by patient's indicating a need for more air, temperature elevation, hypotension, etc.
- Suction would be set up in the room—incorrect; suction not set up.
- Recovery report was accurate and adequate—incorrect; there were many missing details: patient congested, history missing.
- Dressing change was a priority—incorrect; other things were more important.

8. What would you do differently in this situation after having a chance to reflect on it ? (*Reflective skepticism/deciding what to do*)

- Admit the patient personally.
- Get a more detailed report, including vital signs, from recovery and the patient's history.
- Check the room before accepting the patient from PACU.
- Consider postponing the dressing change.

9. How did the beginner get out of her freezing in trying to select suction equipment? (*Chapter reasoning problem*)

- Asked the more experienced nurse for help.
- Took the nurse's suggested actions, and was then able to mobilize herself to take care of the patient.

10. Have you ever dealt with a nurse who was "anxious to give report and transfer a patient"? Describe the most assertive thing you could say to slow him or her down? (*Chapter reasoning problem*)

- Yes. It's always a problem when someone needs to be transferred right away.
- Before you go, I need to get a complete report from you about . . .

11. Look again at the factors that contribute to freezing and at the beginner behaviors that result from freezing. What triggered this beginner's freezing? How did this influence her nursing care? (*Chapter reasoning problem*)

- Interruption in beginner's routines.
- Unexpected event triggered freezing episode.
- Freezing resulted in mind going blank, feeling overwhelmed, giving nifedipine by rote.

Help! I Can't Find My Clipboard

SCENARIO
2

It was my third semester in pediatrics and we were working with adolescents. It was my first day on that unit, and I was really nervous—I didn't know how my clinical instructor would be. I was in the habit of copying everything down from the patient rand card (Kardex) and the medication Kardex. I then always made a worksheet that listed all the hours of my shift and what I needed to do each hour. I put these on a clipboard along with my prep sheet so I could remember everything. I was so nervous that I misplaced the clipboard with all the preparation sheets and write-ups. I was so worried about having lost my write-ups, which had to be turned in, that I became dysfunctional. I couldn't continue with my assessments until I found my clipboard. I had always recorded vital signs on my clipboard. Yes, I could have written them down on a piece of paper, but the only thing occupying my mind at the time was finding my clipboard.

Fortunately, with the help of a classmate, I found it next to the chart rack. I was relying on my clipboard as my "brains" and I was so used to a routine that I fell apart when there was a small change in that routine. I hope that as I gain experience, I will not "freeze" again over something so trivial. It slowed me down. I missed getting to talk to the mother of the teenager because she had come and gone before I found my clipboard.

THINKING IT THROUGH

1. What factors influenced the beginner's behavior in this situation? (*Contextual awareness and deciding what to observe and consider*)

2. What about this situation have I seen before and what is new? (*Contextual awareness and deciding what to observe and consider*)

3. What is one possible explanation for why working with a new population of clients or working on a new unit can affect a beginner? (*Exploring and imagining alternatives*)

4. What beliefs or values shaped the beginner's assumptions in this situation? (*Assumption recognition and analysis*)

5. What is one thing the beginner could do in this situation after having a chance to reflect on it? (*Reflective skepticism/deciding what to do*)

6. How are you influenced by the presence of a new clinical instructor, a new charge nurse, a new physician, or someone in authority who is new to you? (*Chapter reasoning problem*)

7. Describe a time in your experience when a change in routine or something unexpected impacted your behavior in a somewhat negative way. (*Chapter reasoning problem*)

8. What did you do in response to the negative impact? Did it work to get you back on track? (*Chapter reasoning problem*)

9. What got the beginner started in taking some action in the above scenario? (*Chapter reasoning problem*)

10. Would you be able to function without a clipboard or some kind or notes? What would you do if you lost your "brains"? (*Chapter reasoning problem*)

I Forgot How to Give Oxygen!

There was a month-old baby on the unit who was not doing well. As I walked by the room, a nurse told me to come in and watch the baby. She left and ran to the treatment room. I did not know what was happening with the baby but it was sweating, pale, and not crying. I stood there just watching, not knowing what to do or what to watch for. I forgot to put the call light on to get help. I looked down and finally saw a cannula lying next to the baby. I saw that the baby needed oxygen, but I could not remember how I handled similar experiences in the past. I just stood there for a while. Finally I put on the call light and yelled for a nurse. She came in and administered oxygen to the baby. Then I remembered what to do. I took out the ambu bag and prepared for CPR if needed. I think turning on the call light and yelling for assistance helped me put things together in my mind again.

THINKING IT THROUGH

1. What was going on in the situation that contributed to this beginner's freezing for a moment? (*Contextual awareness and deciding what to observe and consider*)

2. Give one possible explanation for why the baby was not crying. (*Exploring and imagining alternatives*)

3. What other resources could the beginner have used in this situation? (*Exploring and imagining alternatives*)

4. What was taken for granted in this situation? (*Assumption recognition and analysis*)

5. In priority order, identify what you would do in this situation and why. (*Reflective skepticism/deciding what to do*)

6. Have you ever experienced not being able to remember something that you had previously known how to do? If so, describe that situation. (*Chapter reasoning problem*)

7. In order to be prepared to watch this baby, what might you have said to the nurse as she ran out of the room? (*Chapter reasoning problem*)

8. If you were confronted with something unexpected, felt overwhelmed and couldn't think what to do, what is one thing you could do to mobilize your thinking? (*Chapter reasoning problem*)

Help! I Can't Seem to Understand What He's Telling Me

My patient was gagging on his NG tube. I communicated this to the nurse, who decided to give him morphine for abdominal pain and Inapsine for nausea. The nurse asked me to prepare the IV for the MS as he drew up the Inapsine. The situation was urgent because the patient was in severe discomfort and becoming increasingly combative. He was tossing and turning in bed, which caused his NG tube to catch on

SCENARIO

4

the pillow or sheet. I knew how to draw up the medication, but I just froze and waited for instruction. The nurse started to notice I was just standing there frozen, so he started talking me through what to do. I acted as if I had never drawn up medication. I practically couldn't understand what he was telling me to do. Fortunately, the nurse was empathetic toward beginners and assured me everything was fine. I was then able to go ahead and draw up the medication.

THINKING IT THROUGH

1. What things were happening simultaneously in this situation that affected the beginner? What triggered freezing in this situation? (*Contextual awareness and deciding what to observe and consider*)

2. What about this situation is similar to something you have experienced before? What is new? (*Contextual awareness and deciding what to observe and consider*)

3. Name one possible explanation for why this situation was "urgent." (*Exploring and imagining alternatives*)

4. What do you think helped mobilize the beginner? What else might have worked in this situation? What are other alternatives? (*Exploring and imagining alternatives and Chapter reasoning problem*)

5. What is one possible explanation for the patient's gagging? What would you do to rule in or rule out possible explanations? (*Exploring and imagining alternatives*)

6. What was taken for granted in this situation? (*Assumption recognition and analysis*)

7. In priority order, identify what you would have done in this situation if the patient had become fully combative. Provide a rationale for your response. (*Reflective skepticism/deciding what to do*)

8. Why was it important to intervene in this situation? What is the worst thing that could have happened if the patient kept tossing and turning? (*Reflective skepticism/deciding what to do*)

9. What were the triggers to freezing in this situation? If this had happened to you and no one helped you through it, what would you have done to mobilize yourself? (*Chapter reasoning problem*)

10. Have you ever worked with a preceptor or an instructor who talked you through a procedure? How did it help your ability to reason? (*Chapter reasoning problem*)

I Thought I Was Prepared

It was my final week of med-surg clinical and I thought I was doing okay. I thought I was prepared. I walked into my patient's room, looked at her and walked right out, saying, "I'll be right back." She had been in a car accident and had multiple injuries.

SCENARIO

5

She was in her 40s. Everything was buzzing and beeping; tubes were going everywhere. I was afraid to move her, afraid to change anything in case I would make it worse. So I walked around the unit repeatedly. Then I paged my instructor. She didn't arrive for a while, so I found an empathetic night shift nurse who walked me into the room. She went over everything. Then my instructor arrived and walked me through everything again. Repetition is a wonderful thing. I will never forget walking into the room and walking right out. Ugh! What a horrible feeling when your mind goes blank and you can't do anything.

THINKING IT THROUGH

1. What was happening simultaneously in this situation? (*Contextual awareness and deciding what to observe and consider*)

2. What about this situation is similar/dissimilar to something you have experienced before? (*Contextual awareness and deciding what to observe and consider*)

3. Were there other resources the beginner might have mobilized to help her in this situation? (*Exploring and imagining alternatives*)

4. What was taken for granted in this situation? (*Assumption recognition and analysis*)

5. When you have a patient with multiple problems and a lot of equipment, describe how you determine priorities. (*Reflective skepticism/deciding what to do*)

6. Has anything happened to you in a clinical situation, either positive or negative, that you haven't been able to forget ? Describe and compare your experience to this situation. (*Chapter reasoning problem*)

7. What did the beginner do to mobilize herself? Why do you think this worked? (*Chapter reasoning problem*)

8. If you were the empathetic nurse, what would you have said to the patient to make her feel more comfortable? (*Chapter reasoning problem*)

9. How might the patient have responded/felt when the beginner walked out of the room? (*Chapter reasoning problem*)

10. What about this situation triggered the beginner's freezing? Suppose this were you on your first night on a unit in your first job. What could you do to get started with the first step in responding to your feelings? (*Chapter reasoning problem*)

I Wanted My Last Day to Be Good and I Feel Like I Failed

This experience happened the last clinical day of my second semester. I had two patients that day. One was 60 years old, a diabetic who had an above-the-knee amputation and spoke no English. I don't remember the other patient's diagnosis, but she was doing fairly well and was able to sit in a chair by her bed. She was probably

SCENARIO

6

in her mid-70s. I had 45 minutes left on my shift and still had to do vital signs on both patients, bathe the diabetic, change her adult diaper, guaiac her stool, and do my charting. I knew I didn't have time to do everything, but I tried. To make matters worse, the nurse I was assigned to was leaving with the rest of the staff for a meeting in the break room. I told him what I still needed to do, and asked if he could do the vital signs for me.

I should have done my charting first and then completed the rest of the tasks if I had time. However, that's not what I did. I bathed the patient and tried to change her diaper and guaiac her stool. It was like a rock that was imbedded into her anus, and she was in pain. She kept grabbing my arm and whining. I felt terrible. I finally got the stool out and began to put another diaper on her. I was unable to do it by myself because every time I tried to move her she winced. However, all the staff was unavailable, so I found an aide to help me. It took us three times to change her diaper. They kept tearing, and the patient was in pain. I felt totally out of control. It was time for me to leave and I still hadn't done my charting. I felt like a total failure. To center myself before I left the floor, I spent a few minutes with the diabetic patient. I stroked her head and tried to let her know I was sorry for causing her such pain. She held my hand and smiled. I guess my problem was that I was unable to prioritize. It was like my mind froze and I just did a task—the bath. I still think about that day and feel bad about it. Looking back a year later, I can rationalize the situation and not feel like such a failure. It was a good learning experience.

THINKING IT THROUGH

1. What was happening just before this incident that made a difference? What was happening simultaneously that affected the beginner? (*Contextual awareness and deciding what to observe and consider*)

2. Which people should be involved to improve outcomes in this type of situation? Which tasks could the beginner have delegated to the aide? What would you have said to the aide if you asked for help? (*Contextual awareness and considering what to observe and consider*)

3. What about this situation was similar/dissimilar to something you have experienced before? (*Contextual awareness and deciding what to observe and consider*)

4. What is one possible explanation for why this beginner felt "totally out of control"? (*Exploring and imagining alternatives*)

5. Which of this beginner's assumptions didn't make sense in this situation? (*Assumption recognition and analysis*)

6. Which was the priority—vital signs, bathing the woman, changing the diaper, guaiacing her stool, or completing the charting? Which would you have done first? How did you decide what you would have done first? List activities in order of priority, and provide reasons for your decisions. (*Reflective skepticism/deciding what to do*)

7. What did the beginner do to gain a sense of control? What would you have said to comfort this patient? (*Chapter reasoning problem*)

8. Have you ever felt you were hurting a patient? If so, how did you handle that? (*Chapter reasoning problem*)

9. What would you say to the oncoming shift if you still had tasks left to complete? (*Chapter reasoning problem*)

10. This beginner said she was overwhelmed and out of control. Yet she just kept doing routine activities without thinking through priorities. Think of a time when this happened to you. How did you get beyond feeling out of control? (*Chapter reasoning problem*)

Passing Responsibility Can Be Positive

SCENARIO 7

One Monday I was working as the medication charge nurse, which consisted of distributing meds to patients, comparing Kardexes with medication records, and informing individual nurses of new orders for their patients. I also had to begin new medication orders. I had done this same job on Friday for about 13 to 15 patients, and with back-up supervision from an experienced nurse. I thought I had a successful day. I only had to pass on the responsibility for about four IV meds to the individual nurses, yet on Monday, there were 21 to 23 patients. I began the same way I had on the Friday before—Kardex checks, separating IV from PO meds on my worksheet, then beginning with passing 8 o'clock meds. By 9 o'clock, I was barely caught up with the 8 o'clock meds, and by 9:30, I was less than one-fourth through with the 9 o'clock meds. I was concentrating so hard on accurately passing meds that I did not realize how far behind I was. Fortunately, the experienced nurse was picking up my slack. Instead of delegating meds to individual nurses, I kept trying to do all the work myself. I felt like I was moving in some kind of suspended animation. It felt like time went by at a different speed. Passing responsibility to other nurses would have worked better.

THINKING IT THROUGH

1. What factors influenced this beginner's feeling of being in "some kind of suspended animation?" (*Contextual awareness and deciding what to observe and consider*)

2. Have you ever experienced a feeling that time was slowing down or speeding up during clinical? Describe that feeling and how you reacted to it. (*Contextual awareness and deciding what to observe and consider*)

3. Were there other resources that needed to be mobilized in this situation? (*Exploring and imagining alternatives*)

4. Why is being the charge nurse different from being a staff nurse? Which duty of a charge nurse would be hardest for you to handle? What are some ways you could deal with this challenge? (*Exploring and imagining alternatives*)

5. What did the beginner take for granted in this situation? (*Assumption recognition and analysis*)

6. What did this beginner do that was effective in trying to deal with this assignment? What else might have worked in this situation? (*Reflective skepticism/deciding what to do*)

7. What priorities were missed? What clues did this beginner get beforehand that indicated that this shift might have been harder than the Friday shift? (*Reflective skepticism/deciding what to do*)

8. What would you have done differently in this situation? What is your rationale? (*Reflective skepticism/deciding what to do*)

9. Have you ever experienced not realizing how far behind you were? Describe what that was like. (*Chapter reasoning problem*)

10. What is your routine after report? What happens if the routine does not work? How do you respond? (*Chapter reasoning problem*)

SCENARIO 8

Help! My Patient Can't Breathe! What's the Number for Respiratory?

It was my second day on the oncology unit. As I tried to get organized after report and checking on the medications for my two patients, the CNA announced that one of my patients was having trouble breathing. His diagnosis was laryngeal cancer and left lung pleural effusion. I started toward his room, thinking what my first actions would be, when my preceptor said, "Call respiratory therapy first." I quickly located the number and made the call. No one answered, and I stood there for what seemed like 10 minutes (but was really only about 30 seconds) thinking I should be in the patient's room. I remember putting the phone down, just standing there rocking back and forth, not sure which way to go next. Finally, my preceptor walked by and asked if I had reached respiratory therapy and how the patient looked. I hadn't even been to his room.

I explained to my preceptor that I hadn't reached anyone when I dialed respiratory therapy. She then said the number I had called was the night number then asked the unit clerk to call respiratory. She hurried off with me to the patient's room. By this time my heart was racing. It took me about 3 hours to calm down and reorient myself for the rest of the day.

THINKING IT THROUGH

1. What things were happening simultaneously that affected the beginner in this situation? (*Contextual awareness and deciding what to observe and consider*)

2. What else would you want to know in this situation? What information is missing? (*Contextual awareness and deciding what to observe and consider*)

3. What are other alternatives that might have caused the patient's trouble breathing? Provide a rationale for your response. (*Exploring and imagining alternatives*)

4. Which beliefs and values might have shaped the response of this beginner? (*Assumption recognition and analysis*)

5. What are your first and second priorities when a patient is having trouble breathing? Provide a rationale for your response. (*Reflective skepticism/deciding what to do*)

6. What aspects of this situation required the most careful attention? (*Reflective skepticism/deciding what to do*)

7. Describe a time when your routines, or what you planned to do, got interrupted. What did you do? How did it influence your ability to think and act? (*Chapter reasoning problem*)

8. It took this beginner 3 hours to calm down. In your experience, when something has disrupted your routine, has it ever taken you that long to get back on track? (*Chapter reasoning problem*)

9. Think of something that this beginner could have done to get out of being stalled in her tracks. (*Chapter reasoning problem*)

10. What do you think contributed to freezing in this case? (*Chapter reasoning problem*)

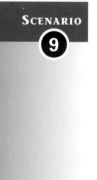

A Float Day

I was asked to float with my preceptor from med-surg oncology to a regular med-surg unit. I had worked an 8-hour shift Thursday, attended lectures from 8 AM to 4 PM Friday, changed in the rest room, and then worked a 4 PM to 11:30 PM shift. This was the float day. I took five patients, and half way through the morning became overwhelmed, behind, and very disorganized. I actually broke into a sweat and felt like I just couldn't do anything. My preceptor was also disorganized. I decided to give one of my patients to someone else, which was a huge decision and made me feel like a failure. Unforeseen events made the morning even worse. The charge nurse called in sick and there were two float nurses besides me. I was never able to feel like I was on top of things for the remainder of the day. Although I caught up, I still felt overwhelmed. That day rates right up there as the worst clinical day I've ever had.

THINKING IT THROUGH

1. What factors influenced the beginner's behavior in this situation? (*Contextual awareness and deciding what to observe and consider*)

2. Which people should have been involved to improve the outcomes in this situation? (*Contextual awareness and deciding what to observe and consider*)

SCENARIO 9

3. Why is it hard to float to a new unit? Why is it more difficult to work with other nurses who are new to a unit? (*Exploring and imagining alternatives*)

4. What beliefs influenced the beginner's assumptions in this situation? (*Assumption recognition and analysis*)

5. In priority order, identify what you would have done in this situation and why. (*Reflective skepticism/deciding what to do*)

6. Describe a time when you felt like a failure in clinical. (*Chapter reasoning problem*)

7. What kind of feelings contributed to the beginner's impression of not being on top of things? (*Chapter reasoning problem*)

8. Have you ever had to adjust your patient assignment? If so, describe what that was like for you. (*Chapter reasoning problem*)

9. Have you ever carried the remnants of an unsuccessful day with you? Please describe what that was like. (*Chapter reasoning problem*)

10. Describe a method you have found for letting go of the remnants of an unsuccessful day. (*Chapter reasoning problem*)

There's Something Wrong with the System

I was going to open a public health case. No public health nurse (PHN) had been to see this family, a single mom with three kids ages four, two-and-a-half, and four months. Child Protective Services (CPS) had visited the family once, but the family needed a referral to public heath. This was automatic because the baby's drug screen was positive. The baby was at least 4 months old, and no one had been out to see this family.

It was normal not to be seen for 4 months because the client load was immense. Clients don't always meet with you. If you set up an appointment and you go and they're not there, it could be another month before you get another appointment scheduled. And this woman didn't have a phone. All these things we take for granted—you have to correspond via mail, and all this takes time.

So I arrived on the scene not knowing what to expect. I thought, "Okay, I need to weigh this baby and maybe do a Denver II. I walked into unbelievable filth. The 2½-year-old was in diapers, just released from the hospital for acute asthma, and all the meds were among the dirty dishes. The 4-year-old answered the door, saying, "Are you here to take me to school?" So I was seeing many needs for these kids and the mom, who said she was not on drugs anymore.

Now, I didn't have a lot of experience with clients who are on drugs, but the mom had shrunken eyes, weighed about 85 lb, and was very chatty. I felt overwhelmed. What do I do first? The 2½-year-old was like a little animal; he was running all over the place and bouncing off the walls. His mother would backhand him a few times and tell him to get to his room. He appeared to be nonverbal, but made animal noises. I found out later that he could talk. I had never seen such filth. The sewage had backed up. The family lived in a trailer, and the floor was buckling; the smell was unbearable. I was overwhelmed on all fronts. The baby was only 10 pounds. She was like a toothpick, little bird arms and legs, at 4 months old.

I visited every week for a while, weighing the baby, and she did okay on the Denver II. The next step was to do a Denver on the 2½-year-old. I never got that far, though I did get the 4-year-old into Head Start. But the main problem was the baby again. She had not gained at all or maybe she dropped a little; it was red flag time. My dilemma was "What do I do now?" I had contacted the CPS worker a few times to update her because the case originated there. They had been out first and referred to public health. So I got on the phone to CPS and said, "This is the situation. This baby has not gained weight, and big time intervention needs to happen." I was not aware of all the workings, so I had called the CPS worker and made her aware of it.

The head public health nurse called our instructor and ripped her to shreds. She arrived late for conference and was very distraught. I feel I did the right thing by calling CPS, but I should have first talked to the head PHN and my instructor. Everything turned out okay, but I felt pulled in two directions and overwhelmed. First, the mother didn't have a phone; I had built a rapport with her, and I thought she was still on drugs. I had to teach her all about asthma. She was clueless, with a 2½-year-old playing with dirt in a moldy, filthy environment. I had to teach all kinds of asthma things. Maybe I got overwhelmed with the bigness of the problem.

I wanted to do this and that—get her out of there. Clean, clean was my big thing. I went nuts over that place. Looking back now, I should have asked the mother to show me how she mixed formula; I didn't do that. It seemed it was common practice among people with limited resources to water down the formula to make it go further. You can get a failure-to-thrive child in that situation. When I held the baby she was stiff. I documented all this. The parenting skills of the mother were nil. Her way of handling the kids was to backhand them and yell and send them out of the room.

But it was hard. I walked into a situation that overwhelmed me. There was so much that needed to be done; I needed to focus on the failure-to-thrive child and then branch out.

THINKING IT THROUGH

1. What things were happening simultaneously in this situation that affected the beginner? (*Contextual awareness and deciding what to observe and consider*)

2. Which emotional responses influenced how the beginner was reacting in this situation? (*Contextual awareness and deciding what to observe and consider*)

3. Give one possible explanation for the CPS response. (*Exploring and imagining alternatives*)

4. Were there other resources that needed to be mobilized? (*Exploring and imagining alternatives*)

5. What assumptions were influencing this beginner's responses to the situation? (*Assumption recognition and analysis*)

6. What would you have done differently in this situation? (*Reflective skepticism/deciding what to do*)

7. What aspects of this situation required the most careful attention? (*Reflective skepticism/deciding what to do*)

8. What is one thing you might have done in this situation to make others more aware of the patient's/family's plight? (*Chapter reasoning problem*)

9. How might economic influences have made a difference in this situation? (*Chapter reasoning problem*)

10. This beginner was overwhelmed by the complexity of the situation. One way of helping yourself out of this kind of freezing is to decide on one initial step to take. How would you decide priorities and what would be your first step? (*Chapter reasoning problem*)

Help! Here's Where I Get It

SCENARIO
11

The next four scenarios are grouped together because of their similarities. They each occur in a community-based, long-term care mental health facility where patients became upset, causing the beginners to feel threatened and intimidated.

A) Last week at the long-term facility, I was talking to my patient, and another patient approached me and began saying obscene things loudly and in my face. At first I was taken aback and didn't know what was happening. A few seconds later I realized the remarks were not really directed at me. There was something in the patient's demeanor that made me realize he was just angry. I finally asked him to stand back, but he continued yelling. I scanned the area for staff and at the same time thought I should be able to handle this. As the patient continued shouting and following me down the hallway, I occasionally answered but then realized it was only making the situation worse. Then I told him I was there to see another patient and if he needed something he had to locate a staff member. He continued to say things and walk behind me. Finally, I walked up to the counter of one of the nursing stations and just stood there frozen. All I could think of at this point was to not respond to what he was saying. He eventually got tired of being ignored and walked off.

THINKING IT THROUGH

1. What was going on in the situation that influenced this beginner's episode of freezing? (*Contextual awareness and deciding what to observe and consider*)

2. What did the beginner do to cope with this situation? What other resources might she have mobilized to help her? (*Exploring and imagining alternatives*)

3. How did the beginner know her assumption that the patient was mad was accurate? (*Assumption recognition and analysis*)

4. What else might have worked in this situation? What else would you have done? (*Reflective skepticism/deciding what to do*)

5. In priority order, identify what you would have done in this situation and why? (*Reflective skepticism/deciding what to do*)

6. What is a realistic worry that the beginner might have had in this situation? What might the patient have done that could have been problematic? What aspects of this situation required the most careful attention? (*Reflective skepticism/deciding what to do*)

7. Have you ever felt like, "I'm supposed to be able to handle this"? Describe this situation. (*Chapter reasoning problem*)

8. What triggered the beginner's freezing response in this situation? Can you think of a way to get beyond surprise that allows you to think of alternatives? (*Chapter reasoning problem*)

B) Once when I was with my client I froze. I had read her history. She had been removed from over 30 locked mental health facilities because of physical and sexual aggression. She had not been violent recently, and I thought we were getting along great. I needed to ask her about her family to write my care plan. I knew her parents were dead, so I asked how her relationship with them had been. She suddenly looked angry, raised her voice and said, "Stop asking me questions." She just stared at me with her black hair falling over her face. I froze because I thought, "This is it, she's going to hit me." But in this case freezing for a few minutes seemed to be the right thing to do. After about 3 minutes of silence, my client spoke again and was calm. After that I tried to space my questions and let her take the initiative in conversation. The rest of our conversations went fine.

THINKING IT THROUGH

1. How would you have gone about getting the information you needed for a care plan given the circumstances of this situation? (*Contextual awareness and deciding what to observe and consider*)

2. What is one possible explanation for why the client suddenly looked angry and said, "Stop asking me questions"? (*Exploring and imagining alternatives*)

3. What did the beginner take for granted in this situation? (*Assumption recognition and analysis*)

4. What aspect of this situation required the most careful attention? (*Reflective skepticism/deciding what to do*)

5. What would you have done differently in this situation? (*Reflective skepticism/deciding what to do*)

6. Why do you think the beginner's freezing response improved the situation? (*Exploring and imagining alternatives*)

7. What do you think triggered the beginner's freezing? (*Chapter reasoning problem*)

C) I had a client who grabbed my arm and, without saying anything, started pulling me to where he wanted to go. His grip was strong and he was hurting me. We were supposed to be going to group therapy, but he apparently wanted something else. He was dressed in layers and layers of clothes and needed a shower. Another client at the facility saw what was happening and told him to let go of me. He did let me go, but started a fight with the client. I immediately fell back against the wall and just watched it happen. I felt like I was part of the wall. I couldn't think and I couldn't move. Luckily, staff members were right there and stopped the fight. Later I read the chart and found out he had a history of this sort of thing. It hadn't been mentioned in report that day.

THINKING IT THROUGH

1. What things were happening simultaneously that affected the beginner in this situation? (*Contextual awareness and deciding what to observe and consider*)

2. What resources might the beginner have mobilized in this situation? (*Exploring and imagining alternatives*)

3. What is one possible explanation for why the client was dressed in layers and layers of clothing and needed a shower? (*Exploring and imagining alternatives*)

4. What did the beginner take for granted in this situation? (*Assumption recognition and analysis*)

5. In priority order, identify what you would have done in this situation and why. (*Reflective skepticism/deciding what to do*)

6. Why was it important to intervene in this situation? (*Reflective skepticism/deciding what to do*)

7. Sometimes, simply taking one step or action can help mobilize you when you become frozen. What is one step you would take in a situation where something surprises you? (*Chapter reasoning problem*)

D) One day I was sitting on the patio with my client and some other clients joined us. I asked my client if he preferred to move to gain some privacy, but he did not respond. I asked if he had heard what I said, but he just stared at me. I felt he was looking through me. I froze because I was actually afraid, not knowing what he was thinking or what he would do. He looked so blank. Having the other clients around scared me the most because I didn't know anything about them or how my client got along with them. After a long pause I said, "It's okay if you don't want to talk, I will leave." Then he started to talk again. I think it helped to let him know he had a choice about whether or not he talked. Setting some boundaries made me feel more comfortable.

THINKING IT THROUGH

1. Besides the look in the patient's eyes, what factors would have influenced the beginner in this situation? (*Contextual awareness and deciding what to observe and consider*)

2. Why do you think this patient stared at the beginner in this situation? (*Exploring and imagining alternatives*)

3. How would you have handled other clients joining your conversation? What are the alternatives? (*Exploring and imagining alternatives*)

4. What was taken for granted in this situation? (*Assumption recognition and analysis*)

5. How would you deal with a client who starts "looking through" you? What would you have done differently in this situation? (*Reflective skepticism/deciding what to do*)

6. What would you have said or done in this situation to help you get past freezing when the client surprised you by staring at you? (*Chapter reasoning problem*)

Look at the Whole Picture

1. In the future, if you encountered aggressive behavior in a patient, name one thing you would consider doing. (*Chapter reasoning problem*)

2. For each of the scenarios, propose a brief directive statement to change the patient's aggressive behavior. For example, if a patient grabbed your arm you could firmly say, "Let go!" What else would work in each of these specific cases? (*Chapter reasoning problem*)

3. What did the beginner do in each of the above situations? Why was it done? (*Reflective skepticism/deciding what to do*)

4. Was the beginner sure of the interpretation in these situations? (*Reflective skepticism/deciding what to do*)

5. Once you decide what is wrong, what is the best response? (*Reflective skepticism/deciding what to do*)

6. In each of these situations, unexpected events occurred that overwhelmed the beginner. When you are about to enter a new situation, what are two things you could do to reduce the likelihood of unexpected events? (*Chapter reasoning problem*)

In a Nutshell

It is important for beginners and beginning nurses to recognize the potential for freezing behaviors when something out of the ordinary happens. But if this happens to you, don't despair. These stories will help you discover ways of mobilizing yourself when you feel stuck. Also, as you gain more experience you will freeze less frequently because you will have found ways to deal with your freezing situations and you will perceive fewer of them as unusual.

You might try keeping a journal about your reasoning, particularly in situations where you become disorganized and have difficulty thinking and acting. Include descriptions of how you felt and acted in these situations. The journal narratives will become experiences of their own and will contribute to your overall clinical reasoning and critical thinking development.

THINKING IT THROUGH

1. Look again at all of these clinical scenarios. List elements in the situations described that contributed to or preceded the freezing episodes. Make a list and tally how often each freezing trigger occurred.

2. In what ways did the beginners cope with and get beyond the "freezing" response?

3. What will you try if you ever "freeze" in the midst of a clinical situation?

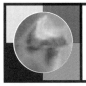

A Sample Mind Map

Step #1

Identify the central themes that describe why beginners feel scattered, frozen, or unable to act. Write them down in the middle of the page. Draw one circle around all of the themes. *Hint: Review your answers in the "In A Nutshell" section. The central themes are: Unexpected, Overwhelming, Unusual Events* (sample: Fig. 2-2).

Something Overwhelming, Unexpected, or Unusual Happens

FIGURE 2-2

Step #2

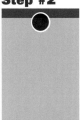

Think of the primary behaviors and feelings the beginners exhibited when they were overwhelmed with unexpected and unusual events. *Hint: Review the scenarios and the "In a Nutshell" section. The behaviors included: (1) going around in circles, (2) feeling pulled in multiple directions, (3) completing rote or routine behaviors without thinking, (4) minds going blank, and (5) feeling immobilized and unable to act.* Write down these phrases and circle them (sample: Fig. 2-3).

Completing Rote or Routine Behaviors Without Thinking

Mind Goes Blank

Feeling Immobilized, Unable To Do Anything

Feeling Pulled In Multiple Directions

Being Scattered, Going Around in Circles

FIGURE 2-3

Step #3   Place the five circles around the large circle in the middle of the page (sample: Fig. 2-4).

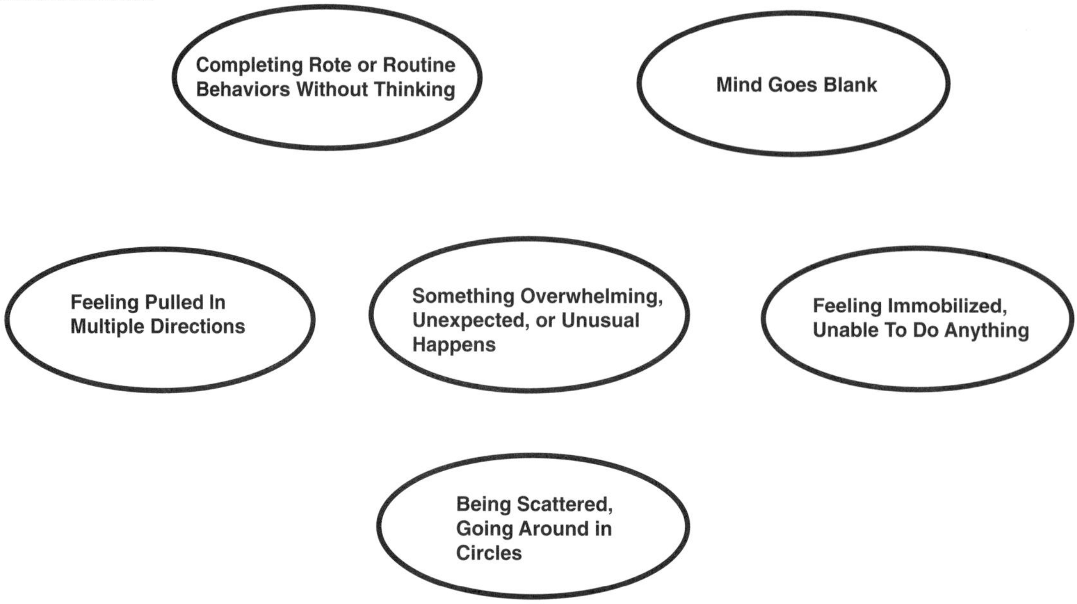

Completing Rote or Routine Behaviors Without Thinking

Mind Goes Blank

Feeling Pulled In Multiple Directions

Something Overwhelming, Unexpected, or Unusual Happens

Feeling Immobilized, Unable To Do Anything

Being Scattered, Going Around in Circles

FIGURE 2-4

Step #4

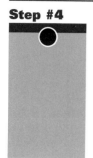

Think of approaches for dealing with the behaviors and feelings written in the five circles. Write them down and draw a box around them. Use a line to connect the box to the corresponding circle. *Hint: Consider what you have tried in your own practice or experience to deal with similar behaviors and feelings. What will you try in the future?* (sample: Fig. 2-5).

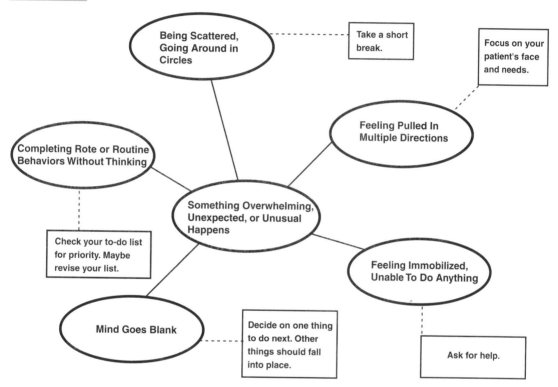

FIGURE 2-5

Feel free to use pictures instead of words. In the remaining chapters, you will be asked to create your own mind maps based on the reasoning problem presented. You may use the above model as an example.

Let's See Another Scenario

Keep in mind the various ways of coping with freezing illustrated in the chapter and in your mind map. Select one of the approaches and describe a scenario when you tried this approach. Describe what you did, what worked, and what you would do differently after thinking about it.

Write Your Scenario Here

Experienced Nurse Scenario

Where Do I Start? There's Always A New Crisis!

I do case management in a public health agency for teenage moms and am responsible for making sure they attend school, have medical care, and use family planning. Donna, 17 and pregnant, was referred to our program by an ER nurse after she was beaten by her boyfriend and three of his other girlfriends. They beat her up so she would lose the baby. She suffered a broken rib and a black eye, she presented with a urinary track infection, and her drug screen was positive for methamphetamine. She went from the ER to live at her mother's house. Probation picked her up for a curfew violation, being drunk and disorderly in public. By now she was anemic and had chlamydia. Her weight gain was adequate but her overall weight was low. There was no record of her ever having attended high school.

In junior high she saw the school nurse weekly, and this nurse reported that she always looked high, regularly spoke of suicide, and used attention-seeking behaviors to get out of going to class. The school nurse turned in a CPS referral, but there was no follow-up. Donna's favorite story was one of being in a fish store with her mother when the mother suddenly pointed to a man in line and introduced him to Donna, saying, "He's your father."

Donna's mother reported that Donna steals from her. Donna attends the pregnant teen program sporadically. Other students say she lies and tries to get test answers from them. Donna's baby was born with chlamydia, diarrhea, and a jittery disposition. Donna chose not to breastfeed. Donna described the baby as "spoiled" and she just let her "cry it out" for hours at a time. Donna reported that the baby "was sleeping through the night" right away. The baby was screaming in the play pen on home visit one. Donna said she had just been fed. When I gave her some formula to check her sucking reflex, she drank 8 ounces. When the baby was 4 months old, Donna held her as far away from her as possible and was rough with her. The DDST was normal except that it was hard to get the baby to smile.

Before the 9-month visit, I telephoned and Donna said she had had a stressful Christmas because she had a grand mal seizure and dropped the baby. The baby had not been seen by a doctor, although Donna had been to a neurologist, started on Dilantin, and had been given a Provera shot. During my assessment, the baby was walking steadily, and was able to pick up a toy but only spoke garbled sounds. Donna spoke of being afraid to leave the apartment, fearing she would have another seizure. I wondered if it could have been caused by depression, crack use, or noncompliance with Dilantin. She was having trouble sleeping and ate only when her mother made her.

While I was there, the phone rang and Donna answered. She slumped over during the call and asked, "What does that mean? Do I have some kind of tumor?" When she hung up she said, "My MRI says there's something, a clot or tumor in my head." No one in the family responded. Finally after quite a while her younger sister said, "Does that mean I get your room?" The mother laughed. I told Donna I was sorry and perhaps it might help to have someone to talk to.

The visit felt like it went on forever and I needed to leave and pick up my own kids from daycare. I told Donna I would telephone the next day with a referral to the mental health clinic, and she agreed to go. On each subsequent home visit, I started with a plan but it got thrown out the window by the enormity of the problems I saw. Before I could get very far with one crisis, another problem showed up that was always bigger. I never felt like I was on track with what I needed to do for the family. As it turned out, because Donna was a dual diagnosis client, the mental health clinic would not treat her. She was referred to the drop-in crisis counselor at Narcotics Anonymous. Her blood clot was real and was from her drug use. On the next visit I did a lot of patient teaching, but I still worry about her a lot.

THINKING IT THROUGH

1. What things were happening simultaneously that affected what the nurse tried to do in this situation? (*Contextual awareness and deciding what to observe and consider*)

2. Which people should have been involved to improve the outcome? (*Contextual awareness and deciding what to observe and consider*)

3. What is one thing you would have wanted to do in this situation if you were the PHN? (*Exploring and imagining alternatives*)

4. What are two more possibilities or other alternatives you might have considered trying? (*Exploring and imagining alternatives*)

5. What was taken for granted in this situation? (*Assumption recognition and analysis*)

6. What would have gotten you started in taking action in this situation if you had been the PHN? (*Reflective skepticism/deciding what to do*)

7. What aspects of the situation required the most careful attention? (*Reflective skepticism/deciding what to do*)

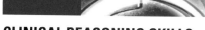

CLINICAL REASONING SKILLS

Comparing Beginners and Experienced Nurses

What differences do you note between the beginners' scenarios and the expert's scenario? Describe these differences related to:

- Details related about the situation

- How she handled unexpected events

- Planning for events

- Ability to respond to complexities in the family's situation

List of Scenarios by Clinical Setting and by Beginner Reasoning Problem

Clinical Setting	Scenario Numbers
Medical-Surgical	1, 4, 5, 6, 7, 8, 9
Maternal-Child	2, 3
Mental Health	11A, B, C, D
Community Health	10
Beginner Reasoning Problems	**Scenario Numbers**
Unexpected events occur	1, 2, 3, 4, 5, 8, 9, 11A, B, C, D
Routines Interrupted	1, 2, 6, 7, 9
Resulting Beginner Behaviors	**Scenario Numbers**
Freezing, unable to act/think, mind goes blank	1, 2, 3, 4, 5, 6, 8, 9, 11A, B, C, D
Feeling overwhelmed	1, 2, 3, 5, 6, 8, 9, 10, 11A, B, C, D
Being scattered and disorganized	2, 5, 6, 8, 9, 10
Feeling out of control	2, 4, 5, 6, 8, 9, 10
Acting in a rote manner, carrying out routines while inappropriately prioritizing	1, 6, 7, 9

 Observe the actions and decisions of nurses you respect.

THE POWER OF QUESTIONING

S o u n d   F a m i l i a r ?

○ I go and ask someone who has more experience than I have had.

○ I ask many questions.

○ I think I should be able to answer most of my questions, but I like to confirm my decisions.

○ Others sometimes get impatient with all of my questions.

○ Sometimes I can't think of what to ask or I don't think to ask.

○ It seems there isn't always adequate time to ask about things I don't understand.

○ Calling doctors intimidates me.

○ I do not feel comfortable questioning decisions made by more experienced professionals.

○ Sometimes I feel bad that I didn't persist in questioning more experienced professionals.

When you don't know what to do, or when you are unsure about something, which of the above behaviors and feelings describe what happens to you?

OBJECTIVES

After completing the learning experiences in this chapter, you will be able to:

- Identify ways to improve your questioning skills.
- Develop strategies to feel more confident about asking questions.
- Learn where and to whom to direct questions about patients' responses to illness and therapies.

- Develop the habit of asking enough questions until you feel all the pieces of the situation fit together.
- Learn to collect the information you need before questioning the doctor.
- Feel comfortable in seeking validation of your decision-making processes.

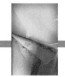

A Short Scenario

Do I Dare to Ask for Help?

I had this nightmare day yesterday. I had just finished report and was about to start planning my time when my patient's wife came to get me. She wanted me to come quick to see her husband because he was throwing his arms all over. I went into his room and he looked okay; he was able to talk to me and so on. I went to ask one of the RNs about him. Then my aide came to tell me the patient in 501 was short of breath and his blood pressure was 198/95. I had to ask for help in thinking through what to do about that, and about the man who had been flailing. I also had a zillion other questions, including the order in which I needed to perform the steps necessary to prepare a patient for a diagnostic study.

I know I asked about 30 questions that shift. I needed to call the doctor, but was afraid he would holler at me if I were not sure of all the data. I realized many things were happening at once, but I felt as though I should have been able to think things through on my own. I felt so stupid. So what if the doctor hollered at me? I needed to call him but was so scared that it took me a long time to finally do it.

Beginning nurses have many questions about what is wrong with their patients, why certain therapies are being used, how to appropriately carry out ordered therapy, what to do when things don't go right, and numerous other queries. Yet new nurses are frequently conflicted about asking questions. On the one hand they need to, and do, ask numerous questions—often 20 to 30 in a shift. On the other hand, they feel uncomfortable about it. They feel they already should know the answers. This could be because instructors often expect clinical students to be prepared with all the answers about their patients' diseases and therapies. Instructors quiz for answers rather than suggesting that questions are reasonable and helping students develop their own questions and find their own answers.

Beginners also have questions about various situations, and when others don't respond, they often do not persist in finding the answers. They feel unable to challenge the decisions of those who are more experienced, and are especially uncomfortable challenging doctors' decisions. Another difficulty for beginners occurs when staff members express annoyance with their questions.

Beginners often generate few possible alternatives about what might be wrong or what to do in different situations. They are not systematic in questioning until all of the options have been exhausted. They do not persist until they rule in or rule out possible hypotheses. When confronted with complex situations, beginners often miss the most relevant questions they should ask or answer (*Benner, Tanner & Chesla, 1996*). Chapter questions are designed to assist beginners in asking increasingly relevant questions.

Beginners frequently ask questions to verify their thinking, but are often capable of answering their own questions. It is important for beginners to discover that asking questions is positive. Many experienced nurses advise beginners to persist in asking questions until all the pieces of the puzzle fit together and make sense.

This chapter is designed to help beginners develop strategies for gaining confidence in questioning.

Recall a Scenario

The scenario at the beginning of this chapter describes a few of the problems beginners have with questions: asking what they perceive as too many to get help making decisions; lacking confidence in their reasoning ability; being unable to develop appropriate questions to focus their thinking; and concern about calling doctors.

Before you begin reviewing the following scenarios, think back to a time in your clinical practice when you felt uncomfortable about asking questions. Write a scenario describing the details of that situation.

Write Your Scenario Here

Thinking it Through

1. What factors influenced your behavior in this situation? (*Contextual awareness and deciding what to observe and consider*)

2. What information was needed? How did you go about getting the answers you needed? (*Contextual awareness and deciding what to observe and consider*)

3. Were there others who helped you develop possible alternatives? (*Exploring and imagining alternatives*)

4. What assumptions did you have that contributed to your behavior? (*Assumption recognition and analysis*)

5. Were your assumptions correct? (*Assumption recognition and analysis*)

6. What would you have done differently now that you have reflected about the situation? (*Reflective skepticism/deciding what to do*)

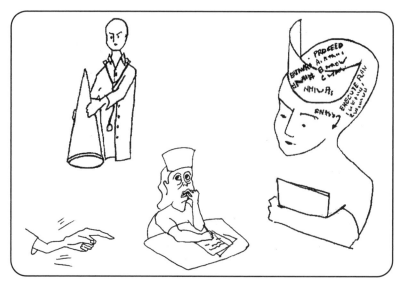

FIGURE 3-1 Beginners have many questions, but often don't ask. They are afraid of challenging others' decisions, annoying the staff, or feeling humiliated. They also have high expectations for themselves and think they already should know all of the answers.

7. What beginner questioning behaviors did you have? (*Chapter reasoning problem*)

8. Describe why the beginner in this scenario might have felt uncomfortable calling the doctor. Contrast or compare a time you felt hesitant about calling a doctor with what happened in this scenario. (*Chapter reasoning problem*) (Fig. 3-1)

Questioning Scenarios

Each of the following scenarios is followed by several questions to help you reflect about what has occurred. They should also help you understand your own questioning behaviors and possibly alter your comfort level about asking questions. Be sure to pay attention to the recurring problems you see and to formulate alternate approaches. At the end of the chapter you will develop your own mind map about your insights and ways to develop comfortable questioning habits.

What Does Waning In and Out Mean?

I had a 70-year-old patient. In report I heard, "She wanes in and out." Being inexperienced, I never asked what that meant. When I first saw her she was in a daze. She would become alert only after I called her name and could then respond to about three questions. At the beginning of the second day she was more alert, and even able to feed herself some oatmeal. Around shift change I was getting ready to leave, and she started getting more lethargic. I was nervous, so I asked another nurse if this was okay. She said, "This is how she is. She wanes in and out. Don't worry." I *was* worried. I kept going back to the patient; she seemed almost limp, different from how she was that morning.

I felt like I was up against a dead end. The physical therapists arrived just as report was finished, and I told them I didn't think she could work with them today. They asked who the nurse was who would be assuming care, and I pointed her out. They went to the patient's room, and the nurse came running back yelling, "How long has she been like this?" I told her, "Fifteen minutes," and she yelled at the charge nurse to call the doctor. The doctor said, "That's how she is. She wanes in and out." The RN said, "I want the doctor here now!" At this point I was just a gopher; I was not assertive at all.

Finally everyone showed up in her room: the doctor, the charge nurse, the float nurse, the nurse assuming care, and physical therapy. But in moving her, the IV had leaked and she had stooled on herself. The doctor repeated, "That is how she is; she wanes in and out." Finally, when pressed, he added that it was the high calcium levels and they were giving her medications to lower that. By now I hadn't charted and I was shaking. When everyone left, the nurse who was assuming care asked if I was okay. I said, "No. I've been telling people what was happening and no one listened."

I decided that I didn't present myself to people so that they would take me seriously. I learned the term, "wanes in and out" is too vague. I should have asked for behaviors that accompanied the waning in and out. No one else seemed to know about her high calcium levels or why she was drifting in and out. I need to learn to trust my own judgment. I should have gone to the charge nurse when the first nurse would not listen. If another, more experienced nurse says something I tend to defer to them, thinking who am I to override that? Sometimes you have to ask more questions if something doesn't make sense. It might have worked to refer to the progress notes to see if the behaviors were described there and question the nurses about any discrepancies. But I didn't do that.

THINKING IT THROUGH

Below are questions about the scenario to help guide your reflective thinking. Answers also are provided to help you get started, but remember there may be others that are also correct. The important thing is for you to think about the scenario and generate as many responses as possible.

1. What events were happening just before this incident that made the beginner realize something was wrong? (*Contextual awareness and deciding what to observe*)
   ● The nurse had cared for the patient the day before.

- The patient had been oriented and able to do some of her own care earlier in the day.
- Others in the situation had not been involved with the patient.
- The physical therapists and the nurse on the next shift were new to the situation and were able to see the significance of the change in the patient.
- The oncoming nurse was assertive about the patient's condition and took action immediately.

2. What factors influenced this nurse's behaviors? (*Contextual awareness and deciding what to observe*)

- The nurse was very unsure of herself. She had not experienced this sort of situation in the past and deferred to more experienced nurses. Though very unsettled about the other nurses' responses, the beginner did not believe she should persist in questioning the more experienced professional.
- The physical therapists, the oncoming nurse, and the doctor were very assertive in responding to the beginner.

3. Can you think of something you could have done in this situation? (*Exploring and imagining alternatives*)

- Ask for another person's assessment of the patient's condition.
- Continue to ask why the patient's status changed so suddenly.
- Do a thorough assessment of the patient's status and review the chart.

4. Which assumptions didn't make sense in this situation? (*Assumption recognition and analysis*)

- The patient's changes were just like they had been on previous days.
- Changes the beginner was seeing were what others meant by "waning in and out."
- Others were correct and the beginner was wrong (the beginner assumed she should not question others' judgments because they knew more than she).

5. Why was it important to intervene in this situation? (*Reflective skepticism/deciding what to do*)

- The patient's condition was deteriorating to a potentially life-threatening situation.

6. What priorities were missed? (*Reflective skepticism/deciding what to do*)

- A thorough assessment of the patient's condition before and during the observed changes in mentation
- Checking lab study results
- Persistent searching for a cause of the observed phenomena

7. What did the beginner learn about how to ask questions in this scenario? (*Chapter reasoning problem*)

- To clarify others' communications and terminologies
- To ask questions until everything fits
- To seek others' opinions when not satisfied with an answer
- To trust her own judgments and to follow up on them

Where's the PCA?

SCENARIO

2

I was working with a 45-year-old male with a T4 fracture. He was a quad with returning movement to his extremities. I heard in report that his chest film showed that pus was accumulating in the pleural space. He had a pneumothorax and a chest tube. He was asking for Percocet or Demerol every 2 hours. I was conflicted about his pain management and felt I should have consulted with the doctor. I really didn't know what his pain was from and didn't know whether Percocet or Demerol would be adequate. The patient responded sarcastically at times, and I felt there was little time to ponder what to do. I had four other patients to take care of.

I noticed that the patient asked for medicine each time the IV machine beeped, and remained evasive when I asked him whether the pain medication was working. He would say, "Oh. I guess I'll live. It's okay." I wondered why a PCA was not used. I thought it significant that he did not report improvement in his pain after being medicated. I probably should have called the doctor, but couldn't think of what to say and I didn't feel comfortable calling this particular doctor. The other nurse was busier than I was and I thought she would really get mad. I had already asked her a few dumb questions. There were so many things I didn't follow up on. I should have been more thorough in asking questions.

THINKING IT THROUGH

1. What things were happening simultaneously in this situation that affected this beginner? (*Contextual awareness and deciding what to observe and consider*)

2. What information was missing in this situation? (*Contextual awareness and deciding what to observe and consider*)

3. What is one possible explanation for this patient's pain responses? (*Exploring and imagining alternatives*)

4. What other possible explanations would you explore? (*Exploring and imagining alternatives*)

5. What beliefs/values seemed to be shaping this beginner's assumptions? (*Assumption recognition and analysis*)

6. What in this situation required the most careful attention? (*Reflective skepticism/deciding what to do*)

7. Would you have hesitated to ask the nurse or the doctor about the pain medication? Why or why not? (*Chapter reasoning problem*)

8. Have you ever felt you did not have enough time to ask questions in a clinical situation? How did this beginner feel about not having enough time to really question? (*Chapter reasoning problem*)

9. What does the patient's demeanor and response to the beginner's questions about pain management tell you about how the patient might have been feeling? (*Chapter reasoning problem*)

10. What difference did it make in this situation that the beginner felt some of her questions sounded "dumb"? Have you ever felt a question you asked was "dumb"? (*Chapter reasoning problem*)

Why Wasn't I There for John?

This scenario took place on the oncology unit. I was assigned to two patients. One was a 69-year-old man with a wound infection and cellulitis of the right leg. He was receiving antibiotics every 12 hours through a heparin lock. The other patient, John, was a 45-year-old man with recurrent lung cancer and shortness of breath.

Jeannie was the charge nurse, and she and the other RN on the team spent the first 30 minutes of the shift discussing why John was a "no code." They wanted to know why he hadn't been placed on dialysis, and why something hadn't been done about his labs. His potassium was 6.6, BUN 156, creatinine 8.0, etc. The night shift had tried to insert a Foley catheter, but they were unable to insert even a pediatric one. I stood by and listened.

The physician who was covering for John's physician came in at around 8:30. He said John had refused dialysis and any further treatment. He said our job was to help the family through the transitional phase. He discontinued any further labs because they had no purpose. He looked at the medications and said there was no reason to be giving the Lasix and to discontinue all the oral medications.

Then the physician, the other RN, and I went and spent some time with John and his wife. We spent approximately 30 minutes in the room. The physician told the wife that the morphine drip was keeping John's pain under control so that he was comfortable, but he might show some agitation. He said he would write a prescription for Ativan and suggested that any family members wanting to see John should come today.

At this time John's respirations were eight and irregular, but there was no gurgling sound. I did a quick assessment, noting that John's body was very edematous. He was a big man, about 6'4" and weighed about 220 lb. I spent a few minutes with John's wife, telling her to let me know if there was anything I could do or get for her.

At 10:00 Jeannie asked if I had given the Lasix to John. I said no because the doctor had said to discontinue it. Jeannie said the order was to discontinue only oral medications. When I looked at the order she had written and the doctor had signed, I realized she was right. Ativan, 1 mg, every 3 to 5 hours for agitation, PRN, was also ordered. She said I should always check the order (and she was right; I should have). I prepared the Lasix and gave it. In retrospect, I know now that I should have asked Jeannie if we could contact the doctor and check the order because the next morning when he came in he wrote an order himself discontinuing the Lasix, saying there was no reason to give it because John was not putting out any urine.

At 13:00 John's wife told me he had been flailing his arms, "staring" into space, and acting uncomfortable, but he was now sleeping. I asked Jeannie about giving the

Ativan and she said, "No. Not unless I had seen his agitation," because she didn't want to suppress his respirations. Again, I wondered why we were not doing what the doctor had told the wife we would do, which was give him the Ativan to keep him from being agitated. I know I should have questioned Jeannie more thoroughly, because the next day the physician ordered Ativan for immediate administration and to be continued around the clock. I didn't keep asking Jeannie because it felt like I was going to her with too many questions.

Around 1400 I went into John's room, and besides his wife there were about seven other women, two men, and a couple of children. His wife looked tired and drawn. I suggested she get out of the room and take a walk, possibly even outdoors for some fresh air. She resisted, saying she needed to be there. I explained that she had to take care of her own mental health and that she needed her strength for later on. Other family members were there and if there were any change, someone would let her know. She finally agreed to go out for a while and later on told me she, her sister, and one of her daughters went outside and did some remembering and had some good laughs.

I felt good about the holistic nursing care I gave to both John and his wife and family. But I was upset that I was not more assertive with my charge nurse. I should have asked more questions!

THINKING IT THROUGH

1. What emotional responses influenced how the nurse was reacting in this situation? (*Contextual awareness and deciding what to observe and consider*)

2. What else would you want to know in this situation? (*Exploring and imagining alternatives*)

3. What beliefs/values shaped the assumptions this beginner made? (*Assumption recognition and analysis*)

4. What assumptions contributed to the problem in this situation? (*Assumption recognition and analysis*)

5. What aspects of this situation required the most careful attention? (*Reflective skepticism/deciding what to do*)

6. Can you think of a time when you didn't question a more experienced nurse's judgment? Recall your thinking and describe how your feelings influenced your behavior. (*Chapter reasoning problem*)

7. Have you ever asked for advice from more than one person? What influenced this action? (*Chapter reasoning problem*)

8. Have you ever seen a doctor tell a patient one thing but fail to write the order? What did you do? (*Chapter reasoning problem*)

9. Carefully word an assertive response to this charge nurse when she said that the doctor's orders were to discontinue the oral medications, not the Lasix, and that you should administer the Lasix. (*Chapter reasoning problem*)

10. When the beginner advised the wife to take a walk, she was closing off a discussion that might have dealt with the wife's feelings. Write a different response that would have more appropriately encouraged expression of feelings. (*Chapter reasoning problem*)

Shall I Implement This Standing Order?

I had a patient who was in her early 60s, 5 days post-op, and doing well. Her vital signs were stable until she went into A-fib, and her pulse went up to about 120. On that unit they had a protocol that stated: "Give Verapamil for heart rate greater than 120." I went to double check with my preceptor about giving the Verapamil and he said, "Wait and see; don't give the Verapamil unless the heart rate is sustained at that rate."

The patient had a heart rate burst of 140; then it went back to 110. She was complaining about a racing heart, and that upset her family. My preceptor said to give the Verapamil, but it did not work. The heart rate stayed at 140. After the family left, the patient's heart rate went down and the patient slept—no problems. I had to give the family a lot of support and feedback to reassure them and to help the patient be less anxious. I really didn't know what to say to them or what sort of questions to ask. I knew I should have been asking questions because my preceptor started talking to the daughter about whether her mother was typically bothered at home when things didn't go smoothly and whether she would get upset quickly. The daughter did say that was common, although the mother didn't usually mention her heart racing.

I flashed on the importance of listening to your patient and paying attention to how they say they are feeling. Since my preceptor was familiar with the routine and the floor and the type of patients, he knew what to listen for and what things to ask the family about. As a new nurse I need to remember that it is okay to ask questions and that I am not expected to know the nuances of the floor. My preceptor suggested it is always okay to ask what the common occurrences on the floor are and what is typically done. It was fine with my preceptor that I questioned whether to go ahead and give the Verapamil from the standing order. Having someone to consult and reaffirm one's decisions or questions can help a lot.

Thinking it Through

1. What is going on in the context that is influencing what is happening? (*Contextual awareness and deciding what to observe*)

2. How did the beginner go about getting the information she needed? (*Contextual awareness and deciding what to observe*)

3. What is one possible explanation for why this patient's heart was racing? (*Exploring and imagining alternatives*)

4. What are two more possibilities/other alternatives? (*Exploring and imagining alternatives*)

5. Which beliefs/values were most important in this situation? (*Assumption recognition and analysis*)

6. What else might have worked in this situation? (*Reflective skepticism/deciding what to do*)

7. What aspects of this situation required the most careful attention? (*Reflective skepticism/deciding what to do*)

8. Think of a time when you were not sure of what to do and you felt reluctant to ask about it. Why were you reluctant? (*Chapter reasoning problem*)

9. Have you ever been fairly certain that you knew what to do in a situation, but checked it out with a more experienced person just to be sure? Did you feel comfortable about asking? Was the other person receptive to your questions? What would you do if someone let you know they were irritated by your questions? (*Chapter reasoning problem*)

10. How did the feelings and responses of the family members influence this beginner's questioning behaviors? (*Chapter reasoning problem*)

SCENARIO

5

What Does He Mean, She Is Just 80?

My patient had lost 50 pounds over a few months. On Tuesday she was feeding herself small liquid meals and was able to move in bed. The next day she was having pain. I gave her some Demerol over 10 minutes. I noticed she seemed to fade in and out. She began having facial tics and it progressed to a tonic-clonic seizure. I had never seen a seizure before. Luckily my preceptor was in the room working with the woman in the next bed. She told me what to do. The patient stopped breathing, and even after the seizure was over she didn't start breathing right away. I didn't know whether to wait 10 or 20 seconds after a seizure for the breathing to start. We set up the suction and she told me to verify that my patient was a code and then call one.

I had trouble remembering the room number and had to check on that, and then call the code. The next day my patient was rigid and stiff. Her mentation was worse, she was incontinent twice, and she had trouble swallowing meds. I asked the charge nurse to do an assessment with me. He said, "The patient is okay; she's just 80." I didn't know what else to ask or what to say to make him understand that the patient was different.

By now the patient was trembling continuously, so I just waited until my preceptor had time to go back to the patient with me. My preceptor agreed that something wasn't right. We went to the chart, didn't find much, and waited for the doctor. He just said, "I'm discharging her tomorrow." We kept saying, "But, but, but . . ." and he just repeated that she was going home tomorrow. Just after that, the chore worker came by, and we talked to her and found out that the patient usually did all her own cooking, etc., and this was not normal. The next day she had a grand mal seizure. The roommate's daughter found me and I thought to myself, "Go get a real nurse," but I went down there and monitored her breathing. An EEG tech ran a strip and it verified she had been having seizures for 4 hours.

It is funny how the doctor denied she was having seizures even though the strip proved it. The nurses said he was difficult to work with and to get orders from, so we got an oncology doctor to come by. It turned out her potassium was high at 6. Her O_2 sats went from 96 to 59 and her BP kept going up and down. We were giving her Dilantin, and her IV had to be restarted. I was feeling overwhelmed because I had another patient that needed to be discharged and one that needed insulin. I went home that night and thought about the fact that I knew I saw changes in the patient. I guess that was good reasoning. I just wasn't assertive enough in getting the charge nurse to listen to me, or in knowing what else to ask or to say. I knew things were not right, but I couldn't challenge the charge nurse!

THINKING IT THROUGH

1. What events were happening simultaneously that influenced the beginner in this situation? (*Contextual awareness and deciding what to observe*)

2. How would you have obtained the information needed in this situation? (*Contextual awareness and deciding what to observe*)

3. What else would you have wanted to know in this situation? (*Exploring and imagining alternatives*)

4. Were there others who might have helped in this situation? (*Exploring and imagining alternatives*)

5. Which assumptions didn't make sense in this situation? (*Assumption recognition and analysis*)

6. In priority order, identify what you would have done in this situation and why. (*Reflective skepticism/deciding what to do*)

7. What did the beginner regret regarding his or her use of questioning skills? (*Chapter reasoning problem*)

8. What question(s) might you have asked the doctor to increase his understanding of this patient's status? (*Chapter reasoning problem*)

9. Would you have persisted in getting someone's attention about this patient's obvious decline? If so, describe how you would have gone about it. (*Chapter reasoning problem*)

SCENARIO 6

How Do You Even Begin to Ask Questions About Such Things?

I was working with a 3-year-old boy who had gastroesophageal reflux. His mom was an insulin-dependent diabetic woman with a history of drug and alcohol problems. Both of her children had the fetal alcohol syndrome look. The boy was developmentally delayed; he was below normal for height and weight, and could not use language. His grandmother tried to play with him, but he would just hold the toy. His mom never interacted with him in any way. When you would do any procedure he would duck his head, glaze his eyes, and avoid eye contact and look like he was leaving. That behavior impressed me, but I don't know what I would have done with it if my preceptor hadn't validated that it wasn't normal.

We went back and searched the chart but no one had charted it. It took me forever to do the charting, so I could just get the behaviors and no judgments in there. I felt powerless to do much more. I thought about telling the doctor and calling social services but I wasn't sure. And I absolutely didn't know what to say to the mom or what kind of questions it might have been good to ask her or the grandmother. I even felt reluctant about talking to the nurses who had worked with him the day before and were there on the unit today. That's what my instructor told me to do first. Then we ended up calling social services and they filed a CPS (Child Protective Services) report.

THINKING IT THROUGH

1. What emotional responses influenced how the beginner was reacting in this situation? What might the child, mother, and/or grandmother have been feeling that influenced their behavior? (*Contextual awareness and deciding what to observe and consider*)

2. What else do you need to know? What information is missing? (*Contextual awareness and deciding what to observe and consider*)

3. What is one possible explanation for the boy's response? (*Exploring and imagining alternatives*)

4. What are two more possibilities/other alternatives? (*Exploring and imagining alternatives*)

5. Which beliefs/values were most important in this situation? (*Assumption recognition and analysis*)

6. Are you sure of the cause of this situation? (*Reflective skepticism/deciding what to do*)

7. Having decided what's wrong, what's the best response? (*Reflective skepticism/deciding what to do*)

8. What questions made the beginner most uncomfortable when he or she considered them? Why? (*Chapter reasoning problem*)

9. Construct the questions you would want to ask the mother if you were in this situation. Would you have been comfortable enough to ask these questions? (*Chapter reasoning problem*)

SCENARIO

7

She Might Get Back at Me If I Question Her

My patient was a 54-year-old diabetic woman readmitted for a non-healing ulcer. She had two prosthetic heart valves, arrhythmias, preventricular contractions, four-plus edema, renal failure, high potassium, and was being given Kayexalate to reduce her potassium. She was incontinent and embarrassed about it. She weighed 250 to 300 pounds, and her Foley was covered with stool. Also, I don't really think she was comfortable with having a new nurse. She was shaky when standing for catheter care. I thought that wasn't a good sign, but I didn't know how to clean the perineal area without her standing up.

Another RN came into the room and yelled at me saying, "She should not stand because of her heart failure." I thought to myself, "Did I miss something? Could she have actually collapsed, although nothing really did happen?" The patient was permitted to walk to the commode if she dangled her legs before getting out of bed first. The RN intimidated me, and I didn't ask anything to clarify her response that the patient was on a heart monitor and we could see any preventricular contractions. I wouldn't have asked anyway, because I feared getting on her bad side since I had to work with her, and I had just been hired on that unit. I should have looked more closely at the chart and thought through how to do the catheter care differently, without stressing the patient. I also could have asked another nurse.

THINKING IT THROUGH

1. What emotional responses influenced how the beginner reacted in this situation? (*Contextual awareness and deciding what to observe and consider*)

2. What is one possible explanation for why the patient was shaky on standing? (*Exploring and imagining alternatives*)

3. What are two more possibilities/other alternatives? (*Exploring and imagining alternatives*)

4. What assumptions were made in this situation? (*Assumption recognition and analysis*)

5. How could you test these assumptions to see if they were correct? (*Assumption recognition and analysis*)

6. What else might have worked in this situation? (*Reflective skepticism/deciding what to do*)

7. What questions would you have asked the nurse or the patient in this situation? (*Chapter reasoning problem*)

8. The nurse was fearful of losing the support of a colleague. What influenced how he felt about asking questions. What about his experiences have you shared? How did not asking questions influence your patient care? (*Chapter reasoning problem*)

9. What questions do you think this nurse should have asked? Which of these questions do you think would have irritated a more experienced nurse? (*Chapter reasoning problem*)

How Do I Give This Medication?

SCENARIO 8

My patient was on the trauma unit following a motor vehicle accident and a superficial fracture of the left ankle. He was able to do his own ADLs. He had two IV medications to be given at nine o'clock, including Flagyl, over an hour period. We were taught we had a half-hour window period to give medications. I asked the RN how to give the Flagyl. He said, "Start at 7:30, and when you're done, start the next med." At 8:15 my instructor came by, looked at the charting, and noticed I had not given the second medication; she was upset with me. I tried to explain that I couldn't give both drugs at the same time, but before I even got that out she said, "Don't 'but' me."

So we went in to give the medication together. Looking back, I could have asked if the medication orders in the records could be changed to reflect how they were actually being given. I let myself get too upset. I never explained to the instructor. I just sat there fuming and let my emotions take over. You don't realize it at the moment when it is important to take a stand. I didn't talk about it in conference; it was easy to talk to other students, but I wouldn't say anything in conference. We are free and open and truthful in the information we share with each other, but it doesn't always feel comfortable to question things during conference. This is too bad, because it makes you feel better to hear your peers say they would have done the same thing. It is hard to stand up and speak out, or to ask questions, especially because as students or new graduates we don't have the necessary experience to back up our points. I could have kept asking several nurses for the correct procedure and then documented those whom I spoke to and exactly what time everything was administered.

THINKING IT THROUGH

1. What events were happening simultaneously that influenced the beginner in this situation? (*Contextual awareness and deciding what to observe and consider*)

2. Give one possible explanation for why this beginner did not discuss what happened in conference. (*Exploring and imagining alternatives*)

3. What is one thing you could have done in this situation? (*Exploring and imagining alternatives*)

4. Which beliefs/values were most important in this given situation? (*Assumption recognition and analysis*)

5. What else might have worked in this situation? (*Reflective skepticism/deciding what to do*)

6. What aspects of this situation required the most careful attention? (*Reflective skepticism/deciding what to do*)

7. What did the beginner do when he did not know how to chart the medication? (*Chapter reasoning problem*)

8. What other questions did the beginner identify that he might have tried in this situation. Why would those be effective or ineffective? (*Chapter reasoning problem*)

9. Think of a time when you were so intimidated that you refrained from asking questions. Pose one question you might have asked. Do you think you should have known the answer? How would you have found out the answer? (*Chapter reasoning problem*)

Do I Have the Right to Question This Order?

SCENARIO
9

I took care of a 92-year-old woman who was admitted from home, where her 65-year-old daughter and a daytime caregiver were taking care of her. This woman was admitted for urosepsis and pneumonia. She had an altered level of consciousness; her mental status had been changing over the last 5 or 10 years, according to her daughter. The woman was still very alert at times but somewhat confused at other times. She was not at all physically active and would get out of bed only with assistance. She wouldn't walk and complained of a great deal of pain in her back and legs.

I was told when she was first admitted that we were basically going to provide her with palliative care, meaning we were going to control her pain and clear up her lungs and urinary tract infection. She was very detached from her surroundings.

Basically she would just lie in bed and look in whatever direction she happened to be turned. She wouldn't ask for pain control and wouldn't complain about pain unless we asked. A problem occurred when the physician decided she was not getting enough to eat, was malnourished, and needed a feeding tube.

I'm not sure why, or how this was determined, but I had to insert the tube. I went into the supply room to get a feeding tube, and asked another nurse if it was the right one. With a great deal of stress to the patient, the feeding tube did go in after several tries. It had curled around in the back of her throat once and the other nurse had to hold her hands down. The woman was in a great deal of distress about this; she was very traumatized.

After we inserted the tube, we checked its placement by drawing gastric secretions, and the feeding started. About a half hour later, we discovered the feeding tube wasn't working. The feeding was going down but was coming back through the vent port. With a great deal of difficulty, and assistance from a third nurse, we inserted a second feeding tube. This was extremely traumatic to the patient. She told me she was afraid to close her eyes and go to sleep for fear of what the staff might do to her.

Up to this point I hadn't known she had been eating typically 80 percent of the meals offered to her, and that it had been documented in the nursing notes. I found this out only after I had inserted the second feeding tube. Apparently there was a problem because the nurses had not been consistently documenting the percentage of the meals she'd been eating and how much she had been drinking. I knew for a fact that the week before she had eaten everything. If I had known there were problems documenting her food consumption, and the physicians were saying she wasn't getting enough nourishment, I would not have agreed to insert the feeding tube. I would have talked to the doctor, although I probably would have made a fool of myself.

I think I was right in questioning whether I had the correct feeding tube, but I was wrong in agreeing to go along with the procedure without having enough background information about the patient, her current history, and the care she'd been receiving over the last few days. Apparently this physician was very aggressive about pursuing treatment. Despite the fact that the patient was maintaining her weight, the physician was determined to get her out of there and the feedings would get her out faster.

The nurses did not like to talk things over with this particular physician. He had a reputation for being very aggressive in treating patients. I did not feel comfortable confronting him with the issue, and there really wasn't sufficient documentation from the nursing notes about the patient's nutrition. The other thing that troubled me was that the patient wasn't really competent to make her own health care decisions but, if asked, would have said no to a feeding tube. No one, including me, thought to call the daughter.

Many older people look at these tubes as something they never want. It was one of those situations where someone tells you to do something and you do it, but later you wonder if you did the right thing. Do you question someone, or do you go ahead and do what they say? I could have told the doctor a blank doesn't mean she's not eating. I could have asked how he knew she was malnourished. She hadn't lost weight, and she had no edema, crackles in her lungs, or abnormal lab results. I keep telling myself to ask questions and not to be afraid to be assertive. That's what I wish I had done in this situation.

THINKING IT THROUGH

1. What events were happening simultaneously that influenced the beginner in this situation? (*Contextual awareness and deciding what to observe and consider*)

2. Which of the patient's emotional responses influenced the nurse? (*Contextual awareness and deciding what to observe and consider*)

3. Are there others who might have helped develop more alternatives? (*Exploring and imagining alternatives*)

4. Which beliefs/values were most important in this situation? (*Assumption recognition and analysis*)

5. Which assumptions didn't make sense in this situation? (*Assumption recognition and analysis*)

6. Why was it important to intervene in this situation? (*Reflective skepticism/ deciding what to do*)

7. What priorities were missed? (*Reflective skepticism/deciding what to do*)

8. What sort of questions would you have asked in this situation, and how would you have phrased them? (*Chapter reasoning problem*)

9. Why was it hard for this beginner not to be more assertive about questioning in this situation? (*Chapter reasoning problem*)

10. What about your behavior is similar to the nurse's behavior this situation? (*Chapter reasoning problem*)

What Lab Work Do We Need?

I had a patient in his mid-70s with a GI bleed 8 to 10 days after cardiac surgery, and a history of gastric ulcers, COPD, and mobility problems. He was really weak and was in atrial fib. He had massive diarrhea with a bad smell, looked pale, had a decreased blood pressure, and had no fever. He was on Digoxin and Heparin. The nurse asked me what I was most worried about and what sort of tests I might consider in ruling out any concerns I had. I had no idea what sort of test might help, so I ended up telling her I just didn't know. The nurse was kind, and she talked me through what she was thinking. She decided to save the next stool and check it for occult blood. That turned out to be positive. Then she asked what other tests might be useful and what questions we might want to ask the doctor, and again I couldn't think of anything.

SCENARIO 10

I felt really dumb for not being able to think of anything to ask. I should have known how to answer the nurse. She suggested we call the doctor and ask for orders for a hematocrit and hemoglobin, and that we might want to ask for an order to type and cross-match his blood. All that made sense after she told me. As it turned out, an upper GI showed a bleeding ulcer, and that was causing the problem. It was a good thing that we had cross-matched his blood, because his hemoglobin was 6 and he really needed blood.

THINKING IT THROUGH

1. What factors influenced the beginner's behavior in this situation? (*Contextual awareness and deciding what to observe and consider*)

2. What is one possible explanation for why this beginner could not think of appropriate questions to ask the doctor? (*Exploring and imagining alternatives*)

3. What else would you have wanted to know in this situation? (*Exploring and imagining alternatives*)

4. What was taken for granted in this situation? (*Assumption recognition and analysis*)

5. How might you test the possibilities out in this situation before calling the doctor? (*Assumption recognition and analysis*)

6. What rationale did the nurse have for her decisions regarding which lab tests were helpful? (*Reflective skepticism/deciding what to do*)

7. Why was it important to intervene in this situation? (*Reflective skepticism/deciding what to do*)

8. How did the experienced nurse think of what she wanted to question the doctor about? (*Chapter reasoning problem*)

In a Nutshell

Beginners should recognize that it is normal to ask questions, even just to verify thinking. Asking questions can result in answers that help you identify what is happening with your patients and helps you decide what to do. Sometimes beginners think they should know the answers; sometimes others' responses to their questioning give that impression. However, it is important to persist with questions until you are satisfied with the answers that you get and all the pieces of the situation fit together and make sense (*Benner, Tanner & Chesla, 1996*). Sometimes you won't be able to think about what you need to ask, but this will improve as you collect experiences. In the meantime, it's good to obtain information from more experienced people.

THINKING IT THROUGH

1. Recall a time when you had problems with questions: too many, not enough, not the right ones. What was the reason for the problem? How would you respond now?

2. Revisit the scenarios in this chapter, and describe the reasons questioning was a problem for the beginner.

3. Do you often ask questions of a more experienced person even though you believe you already know the answer? Would you want to change that, or is that acceptable to you?

4. Recall a situation when you believed you needed to call a doctor who tended to be irritable when called. What did you do? Think of a different way you could respond now that you think about it.

5. What happens when you aren't sure; you need to ask questions, and your charge nurse, preceptor, or colleague becomes impatient?

6. If someone intimidates you when you question their reasoning, what are two possible responses you can try?

7. When you question a more experienced nurse and you are unsure that the response you get is correct, what are two things you could do to feel more sure of answers?

8. When you feel a staff member is dismissing your questions in one way or another, what can you do to ensure that they take you seriously?

9. Which of the scenarios would be most difficult for you to deal with? Why?

10. Are there times when you can't think of what to ask? What is one time when this happened? What can you do when this happens?

Create Your Mind Map

Step #1

In the chapter narratives, identify the central themes that describe why beginners had difficulty asking questions. *Hint: Review the scenarios and your answers to the questions that follow "In A Nutshell." Draw one circle around all of the themes and place in the center of the page (sample: Fig. 3-2).*

① Lack confidence in reasoning ability

② Fear of asking too many questions

③ Inability to develop appropriate questions

④ Concern about calling doctor

⑤ Should know answer

FIGURE 3-2

Step #2 Think of the primary behaviors and feelings beginners exhibited while they felt inhibited about asking questions. Draw a circle around each feeling or behavior, and place the circled responses around the large circle drawn in Step #1. *Hint: Review the scenarios, and your answers to the questions that follow "In A Nutshell" (sample: Fig. 3-3).*

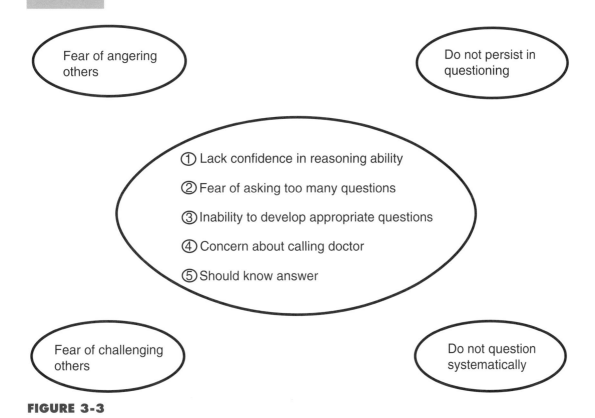

FIGURE 3-3

Step #3 Think of techniques for dealing with the behaviors and feelings depicted in each small circle in Figure 3-3. Write them down and draw a box around them. Draw a line to connect the box to the appropriate circle. Use a separate sheet of paper if necessary. *Hint: Consider what you have tried in your own practice or experience to deal with similar behaviors and feelings. What will you want to try in the future?*

Step #4

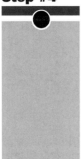

Feel free to use pictures instead of, or in addition to, words. Thoughts, feelings, and strategies you may want to include are:

- Determining your level of comfort in asking many questions
- Gaining practice and experience to increase confidence when questioning
- Asking for help in thinking of questions to explore
- Reminding yourself that you don't have to have all the answers
- Working on a clinical puzzle until all the pieces fit
- Persisting in asking questions
- Working on your comfort level in calling doctors
- Using assertive approaches when questioning
- Resisting being put off by others when you are questioning
- Deciding that others don't always have the right answers either

Place Your Mind Map Here

Let's See Another Scenario

Keep in mind the techniques presented in this chapter for helping you feel more comfortable about asking questions. Describe a scenario in which you tried or thought about trying one of these approaches. Discuss what you did, what worked, and what you would do differently after reflecting about it.

Write Your Scenario Here

Experienced Nurse Scenario

I Just Knew Something Was Very Wrong

I was taking care of a child, a post-op heart patient several days after surgery. The surgery fellow came in to pull out the mediastinal tube, which is not the same as a chest tube. A chest tube lies next to the lung; this lies next to the heart and drains off blood and exudate after surgery.

While I was assisting with the procedure, I noticed that the EKG wave form changed immediately when the tube was pulled—the axis rotated. I mentioned it and kept saying out loud, "Isn't that odd?" I compared the old strip to the new one. The surgery fellow just said "okay." Then he left and went back to surgery without saying anything else. I began my next head-to-toe assessment. The heart tones were more distant. Why did that make me nervous? Maybe more fluid was building in the pericardial sac and tamponade could develop? I paged the fellow who was now in surgery and reminded him that the axis had reversed after the chest tube got removed and the heart tones were now more distant. He asked, "Has the perfusion changed? Have the vital signs changed?"

The pulse was okay, and the capillary refill time was brisk, so I said no. He responded, "What do you want me to do?" I asked for a film and he answered, "The patient is fine. You're telling me the patient is fine. I have to get back to surgery." Click went the phone. But I'm still there with the patient, and I had an anxious feeling that something was not right. The doctor of record had told me everything was fine. I kept watching, kept monitoring the patient. I kept collecting more information to go to the doctor with. I kept telling anyone and everyone. The residents did not know what to do with the information. I told the pediatric team. I told the attending and he said I could order an x-ray if I wanted to. Guess what we saw? Bilateral pneumos, no drop in SATs, no breath sound changes; just air on both sides. That got some attention. We put chest tubes in and the EKG returned to normal.

So the hypothesis was that the mediastinum tube had leaked out into the pleural space. I considered that I might have saved this patient's life. As the pneumo increased, he would have had respiratory compromise. I was not totally sure what was going on. It was not a muscle bleed as I thought, but I did pursue it. I followed my hunch; I kept nagging people and questioning. When you are a new nurse it's hard to believe in instinct because you haven't had a lot of experience that allows you to trust yourself. Still, you should trust your gut and keep pushing anyway. You could save a patient's life. Question, question, question. You have to understand the big picture.

THINKING IT THROUGH

1. What events were happening simultaneously that affected the situation? (*Contextual awareness and deciding what to observe and consider*)

2. What changes alerted the nurse that something was wrong? (*Contextual awareness and deciding what to observe and consider*)

3. Give one possible explanation for why the nurse persisted in following up with so many people? (*Exploring and imagining alternatives*)

4. Why were people not as concerned as she was? (*Exploring and imagining alternatives*)

5. Which beliefs/values were shaping assumptions? (*Assumption recognition and analysis*)

6. Which assumptions contributed to the problem in this situation? (*Assumption recognition and analysis*)

7. What aspects of this situation required the most careful attention? (*Reflective skepticism/deciding what to do*)

CLINICAL REASONING SKILLS

Comparing Beginners and Experienced Nurses

Think about the beginner scenarios and then compare the experienced nurse's questioning behaviors related to:

● Number of questions asked

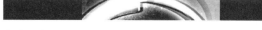

CLINICAL REASONING SKILLS (*continued*)

- Persistence in thinking things through

- Comfort in calling the doctor

- Ability to collect information with which to question the doctor

- Knowing where and to whom to direct questions

List of Scenarios by Clinical Setting and by Beginner Reasoning Problem

Clinical Setting	Scenario Numbers
Medical-Surgical	1, 2, 3 4, 5, 7, 8, 9, 10
Maternal Child	6, experienced nurse scenario
Mental Health	6
Beginner Reasoning Problems	**Scenario Numbers**
Not feeling comfortable questioning or challenging more experienced professionals	1, 2, 3, 4, 5, 6, 7, 8, 9
Needing to persist in questioning until all the pieces of the clinical situation fit together and make sense	1, 2, 5, 8
Feeling like there isn't adequate time to question	2
Feeling that one's questions are making other professionals impatient	2, 3, 5
Not being assertive or presenting oneself in a serious way when questioning	5, 9
Feeling a need to question in order to verify one's understandings	7
Not knowing what sort of questions to ask, not knowing how to phrase a question, not being able to think of what to ask	2, 4, 6
Feeling you should have the answers instead of asking questions	2, 9, 10
Feeling like you are asking too many questions	2, 3

Remember that learning to think critically is an ongoing process.

CHAPTER 4

STAYING OPEN TO POSSIBILITIES

LEARNING TO ASK "WHAT ELSE?" AND "WHAT IF?"

Sound Familiar?

○ I often think of just one possible explanation for what I'm seeing.

○ I often can think of only one possible action to take.

○ I tend to act on my first impression rather than questioning what else is important.

○ I tend to ask others to suggest additional possibilities. I don't see the options myself.

○ Just after report I usually check things I need to do during the shift, such as treatments and medications.

○ Sometimes I miss things when I assess patients.

○ Occasionally I forget to follow up on an important detail.

○ I don't usually think ahead about what could go wrong with my patients.

○ I try to plan the day hour by hour on a worksheet, but I am not good at anticipating how long things will take.

○ On my unit, I am not yet familiar with common treatments, medications, usual recovery patterns, or doctors' routines, so it is hard for me to see what is normal and what is not.

Sometimes it is hard for beginners to persist in thinking of the rationale for what they are seeing and doing. It is also hard for them to anticipate future events. Sometimes beginners are so focused on tasks they need to accomplish that they miss many patient cues and other events occurring around them in the environment. Which of the above describe you?

OBJECTIVES

After completing the learning experiences in this chapter, you will be able to:

● Recognize when you have identified only a few possible explanations for patients' responses to illness and therapy.

● Develop a habit of asking, "What else could be going on?" and "What if [. . .] happens?"

● Identify strategies that help to generate increasing numbers of explanations for what you see in your patients.

● Compare an experienced nurse's ability to remain open to possibilities with that of a beginning nurse.

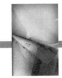

A Short Scenario

Don't Go with the First Thing That Comes to Mind

Not too long ago, I made the mistake of jumping to conclusions without looking at other factors. During my medical-surgical rotation I was taking care of a homeless man in his 40s who was also a heroin user. As I was taking his morning vital signs, he looked just a little diaphoretic and began to complain about feeling nauseated and "burning up." Soon afterwards, he developed chills and started getting restless. I immediately suspected that the patient had developed a fever in response to the cellulitis in his left buttock, which is what brought him to the hospital. However, his temperature was within normal limits.

Puzzled, I asked the staff nurse about the situation and described my patient's symptoms. The nurse told me he was probably experiencing withdrawal. When the nurse said that, it immediately made sense to me. It also reminded me to really look at the patient in entirety before drawing conclusions about the condition and what to do about it. It's important to not just go with the first thing that comes into your head. Sometimes when I'm in med-surg I think only about medical issues; when we switch to the mental-health week, I focus on mental health concepts and do not consider the medical aspects. I see patients as having problems in whatever area I happen to be assigned to work with on that day.

The beginner sees all problems as equally important and can't sort out what to focus on or how to intervene. It is important to develop the habit of asking, "What else is important here? What could go wrong? What should I be doing to prevent problems or to be sure patients are progressing as they should?" It is also important to anticipate how much time is usually required for commonly occurring activities on your unit.

Beginners tend to give primary focus to things that need to be done: ordered therapy, routine activities, and items that need to be charted (*Benner, Tanner, & Chesla, 1996*). Coupled with this, they have limited previous experiences that would help them anticipate patients' potential responses to illness and treatment. Previous experiences can provide templates for some of the possibilities that the nurse should anticipate or look for in patients. This helps the nurse to be prepared and to respond when these possibilities occur. It is important to develop the habit of asking, "What could go wrong? What should I be doing to prevent problems or to be sure patients are progressing as they should?" Asking yourself, "What else is important here?" is a good practice to develop. It's also important to anticipate how much time is usually required for commonly occurring activities on your unit.

When encountering situations in which patients are responding poorly or their condition is changing in response to progressing illness or treatments, beginning nurses tend to close off their thinking after only a brief exploration of possible rationale. They most often generate only one or two possible explanations for what's happening in the situation. Lack of experience with previous, similar situations compounds the beginner's problem with anticipating possibilities when the situation is complex or rapidly changing. Beginners see all the problems as equally important, and they can't sort out what to focus on or how to intervene.

The scenarios in this chapter provide examples of situations in which beginners poorly anticipate time for activities because they lack experience. They do not think of potential problems independently and think of few possible explanations for phenomena. Also, beginners do not sort out priorities, particularly in complex or rapidly changing situations.

Recall a Scenario

Think back to a time in your clinical practice when you considered only one option for intervening or only one explanation of what was going on with a patient or family. Write a scenario describing the details of that situation.

Write Your Scenario Here

THINKING IT THROUGH

1. What factors influenced your behavior in this situation? (*Contextual awareness and deciding what to observe and consider*)

2. What additional information was needed? (*Contextual awareness and deciding what to observe and consider*)

3. Were there others who helped you develop possible alternatives? (*Exploring and imagining alternatives*)

4. What assumptions did you have that contributed to your behavior? (*Assumption recognition and analysis*)

5. Were your assumptions correct? (*Assumption recognition and analysis*)

6. What would you do differently now that you have reflected about the situation? (*Reflective skepticism/deciding what to do*) (Fig. 4-1)

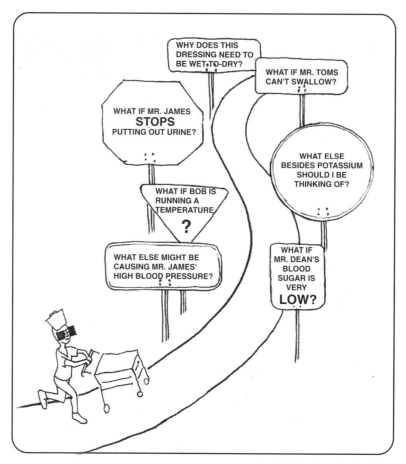

FIGURE 4-1 Beginners tend to concentrate solely on things that need to be done instead of looking beyond the immediate area of focus. They don't anticipate the amount of time it will take to perform tasks, or potential problems that could develop. They tend to focus on their initial impressions of what is wrong with a patient instead of thinking of other possibilities.

"Staying Open" Scenarios

Several situations are now presented for you to read. Each one is followed by questions to help you develop habits of staying open to more than one possibility in a situation, persisting in deriving rationale for your actions, and paying attention to more than just a list of things to get done.

Thinking Backward to Figure Things Out

SCENARIO 1

Just the other day, I floated to the oncology floor. My patient had a bladder repair, retocele repair, and a lot of manipulation. She was post-op day 1 and was getting dizzy. I thought it was the pain medicine; she was a little bit pale and her vital signs had started to change. I called the doctor and he suggested I draw a CBC. Her hematocrit and hemoglobin were low; so we started giving blood. After the doctor suggested what to do and described what was going on, it made sense. But in the middle of a shift it's hard to look at everything and figure out all the possibilities for what might be happening. I should have done more "thinking backwards and figuring out the problem."

You're so focused on tasks—lists of things to get done. Working with my preceptor, I noticed how chatty she is with patients; she would talk with them about things not even related to what she was doing. I can't talk and work at the same time. I have to focus totally on what I'm doing. I don't want to make any mistakes.

In second semester med-surg I had to give 10:00 medications and be finished before 10:30. I was constantly late for clinical conference. I was never good at timing. My instructor would look at my care plan and say, "No, no, no." Then she'd switch it on me. This would throw me off and ruin my whole day. I had to rethink and present two nursing diagnoses before the end of shift. My instructor wanted me to establish goals for the patient, but I viewed nursing as completing tasks. My goal was that the patient not crash while I was there.

THINKING IT THROUGH

Below are questions about this scenario to help guide your reflective thinking. Answers are provided to help you get started, but remember there is rarely just one "right" answer to any question. Try to generate additional answers.

1. What events were happening with this patient simultaneously that influenced the beginner's behavior? (*Contextual awareness and deciding what to observe and consider*)

   - The beginner had to float to a unit that was unfamiliar and did not know the typical routine, staffing, or lab work.
   - The beginner was not accustomed to working with patients who had undergone bladder repair and rectocele repair.
   - It was unlikely that the beginner had extensive experience with patients post-surgery or even with oncology patients.

2. What changes in the patient's behavior alerted the nurse that something was wrong? (*Contextual awareness and deciding what to observe and consider*)

   - Patient was dizzy post-op day 1.

3. What else would you have wanted to know in this situation? (*Exploring and imagining alternatives*)

   - What specific medications was the patient taking, and what are their side effects?
   - Was the patient dehydrated?
   - Were there orthostatic blood pressure changes between sitting and standing readings?
   - Did the patient have an IV going?
   - Had the patient urinated yet? Had she had a bowel movement?
   - Did the patient have cancer, or was she on the oncology unit only because other beds were unavailable?
   - How long had the patient felt dizzy?

- Did the dizziness go away after she ate?
- What was her blood sugar?

4. What is one possible explanation for the patient's dizziness? (*Exploring and imagining alternatives*)

- She was becoming anemic from a post-operative bleed.

5. What are two more possibilities/other alternatives? (*Exploring and imagining alternatives*)

- Her blood sugar was low.
- She was dehydrated.
- One of her pain medications was making her feel dizzy and/or nauseated.
- She had been in bed, not moving for many hours, and she was beginning to experience a consequence of immobility.

6. Which beliefs/values shaped the beginner's assumptions in this situation? (*Assumption recognition and analysis*)

- The beginner believed it was difficult to "attend to" more than one detail or hypothesis at the same time, and she recognized that more experienced nurses (such as her preceptor) and the doctor were able to attend to multiple pieces of information simultaneously.
- The beginner felt she "should" be able to figure out what was going on with her patient. She suggested she should have done "more thinking backwards and figuring out antecedents to the problem."
- The beginner believed her priority was to keep her patient from crashing and complete the assigned tasks, although she remembered her instructor's prompting to establish individualized, patient-centered goals.

7. What got the beginner started in taking some action? (*Reflective skepticism/deciding what to do*)

- Calling the doctor and getting his input helped the beginning nurse zero in on the most likely cause of the patient's dizziness because lab results verified that the hematocrit value dropped from 11 to 7.

8. In priority order, identify what should have been done in this situation and why. (*Reflective skepticism/deciding what to do*)

- Before calling the doctor, the beginner should have taken orthostatic vitals to rule out the possibility of the dizziness being related to the patient being in bed for a substantial period without ambulating.
- The beginner should have assessed whether the dizziness was a constant event, or whether it was related to medication administration, timing of meals, etc., to rule out the possibility of a post-op bleed.
- The beginner should have read the chart to determine if the patient had previously taken the same medications before surgery, how she typically responded to anesthesia, and if she had complained of dizziness to a previous shift.

9. Using this scenario as an example, explain what works for you when you are trying to stay open and consider all the options in a clinical situation? (*Chapter reasoning problem*)

- I talk to myself and silently ask, "What else could be going on with this patient," "What else causes patients to be dizzy?" "Is there anything I need to know before I call the doctor?" "What might the doctor ask me on the telephone"?

- I develop a "What else" list and jot down a few notes before contacting the physician.
- Sometimes I find it helpful to flip through a textbook on the unit to remind myself of "typical" causes of dizziness and to eliminate those possibilities.
- Sometimes I ask myself, "When have patients told me they were dizzy before? What was the cause of the dizziness with those patients?"
- On occasion I ask another nurse, "What am I missing here, what else might be causing Mrs. X to be dizzy 1 day post-op?"

10. Have you ever worked with an experienced nurse who was able to consider more options than you had considered? Describe a situation that illustrates this (*Chapter reasoning problem*)

- Yes, I was doing patient teaching with a woman who had just begun taking Tegretol. I was describing the side effects and how long she would need to keep taking the medication before expecting a decrease in her depressive symptoms. Another nurse sat down at the table with us and also quizzed the woman about her health history. This nurse determined that the woman had a heart murmur, which is a contraindication for taking Tegretol. I knew that it is unwise to take Tegretol with a heart murmur, but it had not occurred to me to question the woman because I assumed that the physician had evaluated this possibility. When I called the physician to ask whether he knew that this woman had a heart murmur, he told me he was not aware of her history. He wrote another order for Paxil, and the woman seemed appreciative that I had called. Later, when I asked the other nurse why it occurred to her to question the woman, she replied that she had previously worked with patients who had difficulties with this same issue and that she asks as a matter of routine now. I appreciated her joining us and now I, too, routinely question patients about their health history when doing medication teaching before discharge.

11. How did this beginner's focus on routines rather than clinical priorities and not anticipating time frames influence the care the patient received in this situation? (*Chapter reasoning problem*)

- The beginner described not being able to "chat" like her preceptor or do more than one thing at a time. As a result, the beginner's assessments were not as complete as those of her preceptor.

Stop That: Let Him Just Go for It

I was in the nursery and not much was going on, so I was assigned to a discharge patient—a woman from Zaire who didn't speak English very well. When her husband arrived at 5:30 I decided to prepare the woman for going home. The doctor had said they should be discharged at 6:00. When I walked into the room the woman was trying to breastfeed, but the baby was all wrapped up, twisted, and not in the right position. He was sucking on his tongue. The woman was giddy. She pulled the baby off when I walked into the room. That doesn't usually happen, but I think she was very shy.

The father was nervous and had many questions. I tried to calm him down, but it is difficult to teach when families have so many questions because they can't focus. I felt

SCENARIO

2

like I was their one-on-one nurse for about 3 hours. They didn't know how to care for the cord, which is the first thing you teach. I was upset with the nurses who had taken care of her, wondering if they had been doing teaching before my shift.

I could tell there was either a communication barrier, or the woman did not feel comfortable learning with her husband being there. She was in pain, had a swollen bottom, and had not received anything for pain. I got her into a sitz bath, gave her hemorrhoid pads, and so on. I didn't really understand what else could explain her reluctance to focus on the patient teaching.

The baby was 5 pounds, 9 ounces, and the doctor had ordered a CBC and a dextrose stick for blood sugar. I don't think the baby ever breastfed at all, because the mother had flat nipples. Nipples need to be worked with to come out so the baby can latch on, and then breastfeeding is easier.

I got the baby to open his mouth; he was a very sleepy baby. It was kind of frustrating because he was a smaller baby, and you think, "Okay, is this baby starting to act sick because he's not eating at all?" He was almost 24 hours old, and most babies are sleepy up to that time. But when it's a smaller baby you do want it to eat and breastfeed well before it goes home. When the baby did latch on, mom went, "Whew," like she'd never felt that sensation before. And then of course the baby stopped and didn't breastfeed well after that, no matter what I did. She was flat and the baby was sleepy. After a while we tried again. She thought the baby fed well, but the baby wasn't even latched on. He was sucking on his tongue. She thought it was the nipple. She was a frustrating patient because she kept taking the baby off, and she was giddy. It was like I wanted to say, "Stop that. Let him just go for it."

You can be sure I went through all the precautions of what to look for. I taught the parents if any of these things happen, you need to call your doctor. The family didn't go home until 10:00. I almost called the physician to tell him I didn't feel comfortable with this baby going home. But the fact was that it was charted in dayshift nursing notes that the baby breastfed well twice during the day. And I talked to one of the nurses and she said that she thought the baby was okay. Because the mom kept taking the baby off, and she was a little giddy, I wondered if she was really into this breastfeeding stuff, and some people aren't. It's okay. Sometimes moms just need a little understanding and encouragement. I asked her how she felt about this, "Are you getting frustrated?" She kind of smiled. Maybe it could have been a cultural thing. She could have been embarrassed to have a stranger talking to her about her body. I spent 4 hours with her, and I had five other babies to take care of in the nursery. It was frustrating. There isn't enough time to figure things out. When patients are only going to be there for 24 hours it's hard to decide what they need, what you should consider, and whether you have missed anything.

THINKING IT THROUGH

1. What things were happening simultaneously that affected the beginner in this situation? (*Contextual awareness and deciding what to observe and consider*)

2. What emotional responses influenced the beginner in this situation? Please address the emotional responses of the beginner, the father, and the mother in your answer. (*Contextual awareness and deciding what to observe and consider*)

3. What about these situations have you seen before and what is different? (*Contextual awareness and deciding what to observe and consider*)

4. What is one possible explanation for why the mother was giddy? What are two more possibilities/other alternatives? (*Exploring and imagining alternatives*)

5. Are there other resources that need to be mobilized? (*Exploring and imagining alternatives*)

6. What was taken for granted in this situation? (*Assumption recognition and analysis*)

7. Was the beginner sure of her interpretation in this situation? What rationale did the beginner have for her decisions and assumptions? (*Reflective skepticism/deciding what to do*)

8. What would you do differently after reflecting about this situation? (*Reflective skepticism/deciding what to do*)

9. How did time influence this beginner's thinking behaviors? (*Chapter reasoning problem*)

10. How might this beginner have benefited from thinking ahead about what might happen toward the end of the shift when first beginning to work with this family? (*Chapter reasoning problem*)

SCENARIO

3

There's a Lot to Keep Track of

I had a patient with a bladder tuck to repair stress incontinence. The tendons that suspend the bladder had weakened after childbirth, so they were resuspended and shortened. The patient also had problems with her vaginal area, so this was strengthened and sewn up. These procedures can cause difficulty urinating. You have to watch for hemorrhaging also. That same day she had quite extensive bladder repair. She had a suprapubic catheter that got clotted. She had so much blood coming out, we had to irrigate it. One nurse said it would just clear out after a while. I called the doctor and we bolused her with IV fluid, but that didn't work. Several other nurses commented that the urine looked pretty dark. After two or three nurses tell you the same thing, you say to yourself, "Okay. Listen to the experienced nurses." Some nurses reminded me constipation is often a problem. You have to be really careful after that surgery to use stool softeners because constipation could obviously interfere with the operative site.

Pain is also a problem, and after the catheter comes out, so is voiding. You obviously want to make sure she voids before going home. You have to do bladder retraining where you clamp and unclamp the catheter for a while. This gives the bladder a rest and helps prevent spasms. It also helps to build tone. There's a lot to remember and keep track of, even for fairly simple surgeries.

THINKING IT THROUGH

1. What was happening just before this incident that made a difference? (*Contextual awareness and deciding what to observe and consider*)

2. Which people did the beginner involve to improve the outcome in this situation? (*Contextual awareness and deciding what to observe and consider*)

3. What is one thing you might have done differently? (*Exploring and imagining alternatives*)

4. What possible explanations did this beginner consider after consulting with others? (*Exploring and imagining alternatives*)

5. Which beliefs/values shaped the beginner's assumptions in this situation? (*Assumption recognition and analysis*)

6. What rationale did the beginner have for her decisions? (*Reflective skepticism/deciding what to do*)

7. What did the beginner mean when she commented, "There's a lot to keep track of and remember to think about?" (*Chapter reasoning problem*)

8. The beginner was getting a lot of information from more experienced nurses. She doesn't say how she responded to this information. What would you want to do about all of the possibilities she described? (*Chapter reasoning problem*)

9. Describe a situation where you needed to keep track of things. (*Chapter reasoning problem*)

10. Other nurses in this scenario were more familiar with typical unit procedures than this beginner was. Have you ever felt as though you didn't know the "routine" on a unit? Compare and contrast your approach to dealing with this situation to that of this beginner. (*Chapter reasoning problem*)

SCENARIO 4

Staying Open to What the Patient Wants

During my first clinical, first semester, I had a patient who was being ruled out for a possible TIA. She was really agitated and said, "I'm here, they told me not to bring anything, and I don't have my purse. I don't have any phone numbers. I can't reach my husband. I can't get hold of anybody." I just stood there and listened to her for a long time. Later I learned her husband had Alzheimer's. He was supposed to be home, but she hadn't been able to reach him or her son. She didn't have the phone numbers of her friends. She was stuck, not having any phone numbers for anyone she might be able to call, and no money.

I went to my clinical instructor. She asked, "What are you going to do about that?" I replied, "Somebody needs to help this woman with her husband." The instructor told me to contact a social worker so that the patient would be confident her husband would be taken care of during her hospitalization. That worked out all right.

That was my first lesson that sometimes I need to think about things and persist. I knew the patient's medical problem wasn't bothering her as much as this deal with her husband. Any day, any one of us could be off kilter—other things crowding our space, if you will. Sometimes you just can't attend to something, so it goes in one brain cell and out the other. So you just don't register it, and don't do anything about it. You're in your own head and own priority, not necessarily the patient's. But it's important to remember to stay open to what the patient wants and to remind yourself to do that periodically.

THINKING IT THROUGH

1. What things were happening simultaneously that affected the beginner in this situation? (*Contextual awareness and deciding what to observe and consider*)

2. What else would you have wanted to know in this situation? (*Exploring and imagining alternatives*)

3. Were there other resources that needed to be mobilized? (*Exploring and imagining alternatives*)

4. Which beliefs/values shaped the beginner's assumptions in this situation? (*Assumption recognition and analysis*)

5. What got the beginner started in taking some action? (*Reflective skepticism/ deciding what to do*)

6. Why was it important to intervene in this situation? (*Reflective skepticism/deciding what to do*)

7. Have you ever felt that something didn't register? Describe that situation and what you would do differently after reflecting on it. (*Chapter reasoning problem*)

8. How did this beginner know it was important to listen to the patient's feelings? What sort of feelings might this woman have been experiencing? (*Chapter reasoning problem*)

Learning to See What's Different

SCENARIO 5

My patient was an 84-year-old woman who lived alone. Her physician had seen her twice in the past 3 months. She had a history of hyperlipidemia, peripheral vascular disease with claudication, and severe bilateral superficial femoral artery disease. Her EKG revealed a slow junctional escape rhythm with right bundle branch configuration. The morning she was admitted, she was in the shower when she experienced dizziness, nausea, and shoulder pain. She got out of the shower, fell, and was unable to get back up again. She was found 5 hours later and the EMS was called. They brought her into the emergency room. At 14:00 she arrived in ER alert enough to tell medical staff what happened.

At some prior time the patient had decided on a "Do-Not-Resuscitate" code status. An EKG at this time revealed a third-degree heart block with slow junctional escape rhythm. She was informed and consented to a temporary pacemaker to stabilize her heart rhythm. She was admitted to the ICU at about 18:00.

Throughout the first shift in the ICU she experienced the following changes: neuro status became lethargic and then unresponsive; blood pressure was initially hypotensive and then progressively rose to 120/76; a bruise appeared on her right cheek and behind her right ear; bowel sounds were present; O_2 sats remained constant at 98%; respiratory rate increased to 35 to 40 per minute with 15-second apneic periods; spontaneous jerks in her right upper and lower extremities occurred; and she had no urinary output.

I began taking care of her on her second shift in the ICU. My initial assessment at 7:45 revealed the following: unresponsive neuro status, pupils slow to react, pulse 60, three-plus edema with 1- to 2-second capillary refill on all four extremities, BP 120/74, temp 37, respiratory rate 38/minute with 15- to 20-second apneic periods, fine crackles auscultated throughout, O_2 sats 98%, nonpurposeful right-sided movements, and pronounced bruise on the right jaw and behind the right ear. At 8:30 I drew a blood sample. At 9:30 the results revealed a significant elevation in her CPK from the previous draw. It was too early for the CK_2-MB. At 11:00 the cardiologist palpitated her BP at 100. At 11:30 I noticed a drop in the patient's O_2 sats by 1%. About 15 seconds later it dropped another 1%. This pattern continued, and the alarm went off. I checked all the connections to the oximeter and the patient. It then read zero for both the pulse and O_2 sats. I immediately notified my preceptor.

When he checked the patient, he pointed out that her breathing pattern had changed. It was now very shallow and slow. He told the family members in the room that it wouldn't be long now and suggested that if they had anyone they wanted to call that they might want to do it now. All but one of the family members left. Outside the patient's room my preceptor reminded me of the patient's code status and that nothing would be done when the time came. At 11:45, I was in the room with my back to the patient. I heard the remaining family member gasp. I turned around and saw the patient moving. I went closer and found that she was actually seizing. Within 2 minutes the patient had passed away.

At 12:45 the same day I was helping another RN with her patient. This patient was the same age and code status as my patient who had just died. Her diagnosis was pneumonia. When I went into her room I found her agitated with dusky coloring. I took some steps to make her more comfortable, as she had requested. Then her O_2 sat started dropping and went down to 87%. I was emotionally drained from what I had just experienced and did not want to go through it twice in 1 hour, so I notified the patient's nurse. She stated those sats were extremely low for that patient. However, her actions for this patient were completely different than the actions taken with the first patient. She told the ward clerk to call respiratory therapy and notify the family of the patient's status change. In the room she took a large O_2 tubing and waved O_2 in front of the patient's nose and mouth since she refused a facemask. Respiratory therapy arrived. By the time the family arrived, the patient was out of her crisis.

In both cases I recognized the patient's hypoxia and decided it was necessary to notify the RNs. In the first case, I recognized that when the O_2 sat dropped, it was the patient and not the machine, which can sometimes be quirky when it isn't making a good connection. I later noticed (after my preceptor pointed it out) the changes in her breathing pattern. In the second patient I observed her restlessness, poor coloring, and low oximeter reading. I felt good about these observations. I was uncomfortable with how the two situations were handled differently, with two different outcomes. I observed nothing was done for the first patient and thought nothing should be done for the second patient either, because in my mind they had the same code status and presented with the same immediate complication of hypoxia.

However, doing nothing would have resulted in negligence on my part and possible negative outcome for the second patient (who was actually well enough to be discharged from the ICU a day later). My preceptor helped me see some of the significant differences in the two situations that I observed but did not really think about. One of these was how the second patient's O_2 sat dropped but then plateaued at 87 to 88%. In contrast, the first patient's sat continued dropping until I was instructed to turn off the oximeter, since it was deemed that it would not get a good reading because her pulse was so weak that it could not be read. Another difference was that the first patient was showing symptoms of a cerebral bleed, either from a stroke or from her fall. These symptoms—lack of movement on her right side, bruising around her right ear, and a sluggish pupil response—were different. Increasing her O_2 and suctioning her probably would not have done any good because there was something underlying that would have prevented her from responding to this treatment.

THINKING IT THROUGH

1. What factors influenced the beginner to think of her first patient when working with the second patient? (*Contextual awareness and deciding what to observe and consider*)

2. What emotional responses influenced how this beginner reacted? Please comment on the emotional responses of both the beginner and the family. (*Contextual awareness and deciding what to observe and consider*)

3. Describe one thing you could have done in this situation. (*Exploring and imagining alternatives*)

4. Which assumptions contributed to the problem in this situation? (*Assumption recognition and analysis*)

5. How did the beginner know her assumption was not correct? (*Assumption recognition and analysis*)

6. What was done in this situation? Why? (*Reflective skepticism/deciding what to do*)

7. What would you do differently after reflecting about this situation? (*Reflective skepticism/deciding what to do*)

8. What did the preceptor remind the beginner of when describing the differences between these two patients? (*Chapter reasoning problem*)

9. What sorts of things did the beginner not remain open to or notice when working with these patients? (*Chapter reasoning problem*)

10. Did the beginner miss anything during her assessments that the experienced nurse noticed? Please contrast the two nurses' assessments. How did the experienced nurse's assessment influence her actions? (*Chapter reasoning problem*)

SCENARIO 6

Seeing What Will Happen

I was working with a 13-year-old white male patient on the children's unit of an acute inpatient psychiatric hospital. The child was admitted for pyromania, inappropriate acting out (i.e., physically, sexually, and verbally), rule out Tourette's syndrome, and sexual abuse. It was my first day there, and when the nursing staff met me and realized I was African-American, they gave me the option of an assignment with another patient because the child had demonstrated behaviors that suggested racial intolerance of African-Americans. However, I decided that this patient would be a challenge and a great opportunity for both of us.

The patient was from a small town that is 99% white, and I figured his impressions of African-Americans probably came from the media and others who also may have had little experience with African-Americans. I figured if I could get close to this patient, I would have an opportunity to change his perception of African-Americans to some degree.

On both days I was there, I followed the patient to school and groups and observed a great deal of the inappropriate behavior he was admitted for. I redirected the behavior each time. Within a short time, I began to gain his confidence and he verbalized personal issues openly. The patient often looked to me for approval and/or disapproval before making a move.

By noon of the first day, I was talking to the patient in his room and observed racial slurs about African-Americans on the doors, walls, and furniture. The staff members confirmed that the patient had written the slurs and previously had been required to remove them. So I instructed him to wash the slurs off the walls.

While he washed, I began asking him questions. After each response, I would give a positive view or provide a different perspective. For example, the patient had written, "Snoop Doggy Dog sucks. Rap music sucks." The patient denied writing this phrase, but admitted he did not like rap music. I told the patient that I dislike listening to heavy metal, but that I do not dislike the people who sing it or the people who like it.

As my conversation continued, I asked the patient to name some African-Americans he admired. The patient named some sports figures and then said that he admired me. I ended up feeling that maybe, if only for the 2 days that I worked with him, I touched something in him that helped him to realize that his view of African-Americans was wrong. I did not expect long-term change in just 2 days, but I hoped that the patient would not forget the positive experience he had with me. This was basically a good kid with poor guidance.

THINKING IT THROUGH

1. What emotional responses influenced how the beginner reacted in this situation? (*Contextual awareness and deciding what to observe and consider*)

2. What is one possible explanation for why the child responded as he did? (*Exploring and imagining alternatives*)

3. Which beliefs/values shaped the beginner's assumptions in this situation? (*Assumption recognition and analysis*)

4. What would you have done differently in this situation? (*Reflective skepticism/deciding what to do*)

5. What influenced this beginner to volunteer to work with this child? (*Chapter reasoning problem*)

6. In what ways did this beginner seek input from the staff while working with this child? What two possibilities did the staff help this beginner consider? (*Chapter reasoning problem*)

7. Why did the staff suggest that it might not be wise for this beginner to work with a child who came from a small town, expressed anger toward African-Americans, was acting out sexually and physically, and could have both Tourette's syndrome and a history of sexual abuse? (*Chapter reasoning problem*)

What Else Should I Chart?

I was working on the trauma unit. It was toward the end of my second semester and I had four patients. One was a drug abuser who had multiple gunshot wounds suffered during a drug deal gone bad. He had five bullet wounds, two in the left leg, two in the chest, and one in his upper left arm. He was on a PCA pump and an antibiotic, and he needed to have the dressing changed on each of his wounds. During report, I was told that the previous shift was unable to change his dressings and that I was to try to change them. When I entered the patient's room, he said he didn't want to be bothered and I should leave the room, so I did. After I did the morning assessments on my other patients, the nurse in charge of his care told me he had not let anyone change his dressing in three shifts, and if he still did not cooperate I shouldn't be too concerned. The patient was going to call the doctor and have himself discharged. I had three other patients, so I didn't worry about it. In the nursing notes I wrote that the patient refused nursing care. I did not give it a second thought.

Around noon, when the clinical instructor came by to check out my charting, she asked why I had not charted the assessment on this patient. I explained that he had refused care, and I had reported that in the nursing progress notes. The instructor then asked if, while talking to him, I had noticed whether he was alert and oriented or whether his breathing was labored. She then asked if I had noticed the condition of his skin, whether I had checked his urinal for color and condition, and whether or not he was eating.

I soon realized why the instructor was asking me all these questions. Although the patient had refused a dressing change, I could have charted his respiration rate, skin condition, intake and output, and many other things about the patient. The instructor was not being hard on me. She was only pointing out that sometimes you have to work with what you have; you never give up. I had taken the easy way out. Later, the doctor came in and told the patient that if he was not going to let the nurses change his dressings, he was to be discharged immediately. The patient decided to cooperate. I learned a valuable lesson that day that I will never forget, "Don't take the easy way out no matter how difficult the patient is."

THINKING IT THROUGH

1. What factors influenced the beginner's behavior in this situation? What behaviors and feelings that the patient communicated affected the beginner's actions? (*Contextual awareness and deciding what to observe and consider*)

2. What about this situation have you seen before and what is different? (*Contextual awareness and deciding what to observe and consider*)

3. What else would you have wanted to know in this situation? (*Exploring and imaging alternatives*)

4. What was taken for granted in this situation? (*Assumption recognition and analysis*)

5. What would you have done differently after reflecting about this situation? (*Reflective skepticism/deciding what to do*)

6. What priorities were missed? (*Reflective skepticism/deciding what to do*)

7. Describe a time in your experience when a patient refused treatment. What did you do? How was what you did different from/the same as the beginner's behavior in this scenario? What would you do differently now? (*Chapter reasoning problem*)

8. What did the instructor help this beginner understand about assessments? (*Chapter reasoning problem*)

Was it Really an Air Bubble?

I walked into the nursery, and the patient was cherry pink and on a ventilator. The room was subdued, the lights were down, and the room was calm. When report started it got a little noisy, but the patient did not respond with agitation when the noise level increased. The nurse I was getting report from was new. She said the infant had a PaO_2 of 110. We repeated it twice, and suspected there were air bubbles in the specimen, so we didn't do anything.

The first thing I did was assess the oxygenation because the report did not fit with the clinical picture. Something else had to be going on. The baby, which was preterm, was 100% oxygenated, as high as it can go. Preterm babies rarely get 100% oxygenated; they are usually in the low 90s or high 80s, which is where you want them. The ventilator was on room air, 21%. It just didn't fit, and the baby was bright red. I called respiratory and said, "Something just doesn't fit." I asked if they could just check out the system for me. They found the system was hooked to the wall unit on 100% oxygen instead of the ventilator blender that was on room air. So, for 5 hours they had been giving 100% oxygen. The baby did fine, although I was worried about his eyes.

THINKING IT THROUGH

1. What was going on in the situation that was influencing what was happening? (*Contextual awareness and deciding what to observe and consider*)

2. What else did this beginner need to know? What information was missing? (*Contextual awareness and deciding what to observe and consider*)

3. What is one possible explanation for why the nurse called respiratory to check the system? (*Exploring and imagining alternatives*)

4. Were there others who might have helped develop more alternatives? (*Exploring and imagining alternatives*)

5. What was taken for granted in this situation? (*Assumption recognition and analysis*)

6. Which assumptions contributed to the problem in this situation? (*Assumption recognition and analysis*)

7. What rationale did the nurse have for her decisions and questions? (*Reflective skepticism/deciding what to do*)

8. In priority order, identify what should have been done in this situation and why. (*Reflective skepticism/deciding what to do*)

9. Why was the experienced nurse concerned about the baby's eyes? (*Chapter reasoning problem*)

10. What conclusion did the new nurse make about why the PaO$_2$ was 110? What other explanations did the experienced nurse explore? (*Chapter reasoning problem*)

SCENARIO 9

Staying Open to Other Interpretations

I was working with my one-to-one patient, a paranoid schizophrenic in her early 20s. She went home from the locked psychiatric facility twice each week to visit her family. One day I asked her what she most enjoyed about going home, and she responded, "Cigarettes and scalloped potatoes." Her voice was flat. I concluded that food and cigarettes were the most important things in her life and that she did not really value relationships with her family. I discussed this with a classmate, who suggested that maybe the family didn't know how to talk with my client, or maybe they felt nervous around her because some of her mannerisms are a bit odd. She sometimes postures and put her hands in peculiar positions. I hadn't considered that possibility. Then I talked with the staff. They felt my patient was just very literal and suggested that in order to get an answer that wasn't overly literal, my questions needed to be more direct, such as: "What do you value about your visits with your sister?" The staff also reminded me that schizophrenics almost always talk in a flat voice tone, without a lot of emotion. I learned that it's important to seek out several reasons for a patient's behavior before drawing a conclusion.

THINKING IT THROUGH

1. What else did this beginner need to know? What information was missing? (*Contextual awareness and deciding what to observe and consider*)

2. Were there other resources that needed to be mobilized? (*Contextual awareness and deciding what to observe and consider*)

3. What did the beginner take for granted? (*Assumption recognition and analysis*)

4. How could the beginner have backed up or eliminated her assumption about what the patient most valued? (*Assumption recognition and analysis*)

5. What aspects of this situation required the most careful attention? (*Reflective skepticism/deciding what to do*)

6. What got the beginner started in taking some action to reconsider his or her conclusions? Why did it help to talk with her classmate and the staff? (*Reflective skepticism/deciding what to do*)

7. Describe a time when you considered only one explanation for a patient's behavior. What are two things you could have done to extend your considerations? (*Chapter reasoning problem*)

8. What else would you have done to elicit the patient's reaction to her home visit and family? (*Chapter reasoning problem*)

What Else Could Change in Just One Day?

My patient's potassium chloride IV was running out when I came on shift. She was an elderly woman who had burns on her arms from an accident in her kitchen. Her potassium had been within normal limits the day before. I was in the nursing station getting a new IV bag and labeling the bag and writing down the time to change it. It was the first time I ever changed an IV bag because I had just been checked off on this in the lab on campus the week before. The RN who was taking care of the patient came running down the hall to tell me the patient's potassium level was too high and we had to call the doctor for a new order. The patient had a heart condition and took Lasix. There was also some problem with her renal function not being all that great. I didn't consider the possibility that the potassium level could change that much in just one day. But after that experience, I learned the importance of checking the lab values constantly.

Thinking it Through

1. What about this situation have you seen before and what is different? (*Contextual awareness and deciding what to observe and consider*)

2. What is one thing you could have done? (*Exploring and imagining alternatives*)

3. What did the beginner take for granted in this situation? (*Assumption recognition and analysis*)

4. Why was it important to intervene in this situation? (*Reflective skepticism/deciding what to do*)

5. What would you have done differently after reflecting about this situation? (*Reflective skepticism/deciding what to do*)

6. This beginner didn't think about what could go wrong. Describe a time that happened to you. How did that experience change your behavior? (*Chapter reasoning problem*)

7. What details did this beginner forget to follow up on as she was focused on changing the IV? (*Chapter reasoning problem*)

I Should Have Known

I was being oriented to the cardiac post-intensive care unit. I had been taking care of only one patient for the first week. This evening I said, "I want two patients." So they gave me the ICU transfer and someone who was a piece of cake. I quote, "a piece of cake." The transfer patient had six or eight lines going in and I was confused, but that patient ended up being okay. I mean it was really confusing to see all these tubes going in and out, but he didn't have any arrhythmias or anything and he slept most of the shift. But my "piece of cake" patient went into v-tach, which, you know, is life-threatening. It wasn't just a few beats; it was a 25 beat run. It was going across the monitor. And I had no idea what to do. I heard the monitor tech scream, "The patient's in v-tach." And I'm going, "Now what?" Before I could even go through the motions of figuring what to do, my preceptor was already in there giving the lidocaine. I know what to do now, and I know where the lidocaine is. Ever since then, I figure out what's commonly recurring on any unit and I begin asking, "What if . . . ," thinking of things that could go wrong and what I'd do. I spend the time driving to work doing the "what if" thinking.

SCENARIO

11

THINKING IT THROUGH

1. What about this situation influenced this beginner's behaviors? (*Contextual awareness and deciding what to observe and consider*)

2. What would you have done differently after reflecting on the situation? (*Exploring and imagining alternatives*)

3. What was being taken for granted in this situation? (*Assumption recognition and analysis*)

4. What aspects of this situation required the most careful attention? (*Reflective skepticism/deciding what to do*)

5. This beginner decided to deliberately rehearse certain possible situations. What is the rationale for doing that? (*Chapter reasoning problem*)

6. This beginner focused on the routine of admitting the patient and missed an important priority. What else might the beginner have tried or considered? (*Chapter reasoning problem*)

7. What are commonly occurring events on the unit where you are working? Have you thought through what you would do if these events occurred? (*Chapter reasoning problem*)

Staying Open to the Patient's Feelings

This scenario has to do with allocating and prioritizing my time. My community health caseload included a very elderly woman and her elderly daughter, a young mother ("A") with a toddler, and another young mother ("B"). Mother "B" was several months pregnant and had not had any prenatal care. She had three other children under 4 years old, including an infant who was hospitalized last fall for failure to thrive, a toddler who was hospitalized at about the same time for asthma, and another little boy who seemed to be okay. CPS and Public Health were involved during these hospitalizations, and the client felt very threatened and negative as a result of her perceptions of CPS's opinion of her mothering. I was delighted when she allowed me to visit, and I knew I would have to deal very carefully with her. Neither of these young mothers had a telephone, so during the previous week's visit, I scheduled appointments for the following Thursday afternoon, with no time specified.

On that day, I asked my PHN to visit mother "A," a high-risk case, at 3:00. Then I went to see my elderly ladies. They told me they were about to lose their rented home, so I spent some time when I got back to the office locating and contacting some referrals to help them get housing and possibly housing assistance. That didn't leave enough time to visit mother "B" before my scheduled visit to mother "A" with my PHN. Since she didn't have a telephone, I couldn't let mother "B" know about the change in plan. When I left the office for the day, I dropped by mother "B's" apartment to apologize for missing our appointment and to reschedule. She was furious that I hadn't come, said she'd had things to do but had been waiting around all day for me to come, and said she didn't think she wanted me or anybody to come any more. Since it was 6:00 pm and she was in the process of feeding her children, I chose not to defend myself or continue the discussion, but I did call my PHN the next day to let her know what had happened.

I felt really bad about this situation. I think I failed to take into consideration what a "brittle" client she was and neglected to find alternative courses of action that would have allowed me time to either make my scheduled visit with her or at least let her know earlier that I would not be coming. Maybe I should have recognized the situation earlier so I could have stopped by after my visit with the elderly clients to reschedule our visit before I even got into the afternoon.

SCENARIO
12

THINKING IT THROUGH

1. What was important and what wasn't in this situation? (*Contextual awareness and deciding what to observe and consider*)

2. What factors influenced this beginner's behavior in this situation? (*Contextual awareness and deciding what to observe and consider*)

3. What is one thing you could have done in this situation? (*Exploring and imagining alternatives*)

4. What are two other possibilities/alternatives? (*Exploring and imagining alternatives*)

5. Which beliefs/values shaped the beginner's assumptions in this situation? (*Assumption recognition and analysis*)

6. In what way did assumptions influence this situation? (*Assumption recognition and analysis*)

7. In priority order, identify what you would have done in this situation and why? (*Reflective skepticism/deciding what to do*)

8. How might the outcome have been different if the beginner had imagined a possible response in the mother who waited for her all day? (*Chapter reasoning problem*)

9. What feelings might Mother "B" have been experiencing that explained why she was angry with the beginner? Why was it good that the beginner did not "defend" herself? (*Chapter reasoning problem*)

10. Have you ever failed to anticipate how long a visit or a task would take? Describe the similarities with this situation and your own. (*Chapter reasoning problem*)

11. What did the beginner mean when she commented that only one possible action or alternative came to her mind in this situation? Has that ever happened to you? (*Chapter reasoning problem*)

In a Nutshell

Beginners tend to focus on tasks they need to accomplish during a shift, such as administering medications, performing assessments, and charting. Because each task seems equally important, they have difficulty prioritizing. Additionally, they have little experience with procedures and find it difficult to anticipate how long they will take. It's also hard for beginners to anticipate possible patient responses to disease and therapies because they have few patterns for this from past experiences.

To overcome these obstacles, you should try to obtain sustained experience in the same environment and stay on the same shift on the same unit if possible. You can build your experiences with commonly occurring events, such as the medications commonly ordered, the doctor's usual ordered treatments, patients' common responses, and the commonly occurring diseases or surgeries occurring on the unit. Also, it helps to be very deliberate in asking yourself questions such as:

- "What if . . . ?"
- "What could go wrong?"
- "What happens pretty often in these cases?"
- "What are some common problems with this medication?"
- "If the patient [. . .], what will I do?"

It may help to keep a journal of experiences that stand out for you as you practice. You might ask more experienced nurses on the unit to help you anticipate things that happen often on the unit. Also, more experienced nurses might assist you by reviewing commonly recurring events and responses to these events.

THINKING IT THROUGH

1. Review the scenarios in this chapter. How would anticipating events have helped the beginners? How would it have helped to plan time more carefully?

2. Choose two scenarios and ask some "what if" questions, trying to anticipate what might have happened in the future. List what you would have done.

3. Choose two scenarios and make a list of what else might explain what was happening.

4. Think of two scenarios from your own experiences in the last month. Think of as many possible explanations for what you were seeing in your patients' responses to therapies and to their diseases.

5. What is your usual routine after report? How could you expand this routine to remain open to what is happening with patients?

6. While starting on your assessments, if a patient said something you didn't anticipate, would it be hard for you to change your focus from assessments? What might you do to help you change your focus?

7. On your unit, what are the commonly occurring medications, treatments, doctors' orders, surgeries, diagnoses, and lab studies? How does a knowledge of this help you anticipate what might happen in the future?

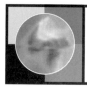

*Create Your Mind Map**

Step #1

Identify factors that contributed to the beginner's behaviors and feelings in this scenario. Write down these factors and draw a circle around them. *Hint: Review the scenarios and your answers to the questions that follow "In a Nutshell."*

Step #2

Think of the behaviors and feelings beginners exhibit when they don't explore options. Write them down and draw a circle around each feeling or behavior. Place the circles around the one drawn in Step #1.

Step #3

Think of approaches for coping with the behaviors or feelings described. Write them down and draw a box around them. Then draw a line to connect the box to the appropriate circle. *Hint: Consider what you have tried in your own practice or experience to deal with similar behaviors and feelings. What will you want to try in the future? Coping approaches may include:*

- Anticipating possible events
- Practicing responses to "what if" questions
- Noting what is commonly occurring
- Generating likely possibilities
- Recognizing what is outside the norm with a given patient

Step #4

You may also use pictures to portray the chapter's central theme and ways of coping with the scenario problems.

---

*For Steps 1 and 2, use a separate sheet of paper if necessary.

Place Your Mind Map Here

Let's See Another Scenario

This chapter looked at ways to help beginners remember to consider "what else" and "what if" questions in clinical situations. Select one of these approaches, and describe a scenario in which you tried or thought about using this approach. Discuss what you did, what worked, and what you would have done differently after thinking about it.

In your future clinical experiences, whenever you feel stuck in considering just one option, alternative, or course of action, think back to this scenario. You also may consider adding it to your journal.

Write Your Scenario Here

Experienced Nurse Scenario

The Value of Staying Open

Recently I received an 82-year-old woman, post-op day 1. In report, I learned that she had a coronary artery bypass graph, CABG, and mitral valve replacement. She had quite a long history of congestive heart failure, and the nurse had told me she had scattered crackles throughout her lung fields. The physician had ordered Lasix, a common diuretic. Many people who come out of surgery are what we call "wet"—they get edematous. Sometimes their lung fields are pretty full. So we need to get that extra water off quickly. Yet, one of the things Lasix does is deplete volume and lower blood pressure, mostly because of the depletion; but it also vasodilates you. So, according to report, when they gave her 40 Lasix, her blood pressure dropped into the 70s; her normal blood pressure was in the low 100s. When blood pressure becomes that low, everyone is concerned. Sometimes we give medications to counteract it, or we increase it with pressors. But that wasn't the case with this patient.

The ICU nurse told the physician, "You'd better write an order to cover this low blood pressure because she's chronically low." So he did. He said to call for a blood pressure of anything less than 80. This is systolic blood pressure. I wouldn't mind a diastolic at 80. The patient had a Foley catheter and produced about 450 cc urine while in the ICU and on our shift. This isn't a huge amount for having 40 of Lasix.

The patient also had a valve repair. We wanted to keep her fairly anticoagulated because new mechanical valves tend to make little clots, so she was on heparin drip. We have protocol that dictates how anticoagulated patients should be, and it said maintain infusion to maintain PTT of 35 to 45. The patient was in range. She was in normal sinus rhythm, with some premature ventricular contractions, but nothing serious. Also, I was told in report that she had an ejection fraction of 25%; when the ventricles contract, that's how much they push up. Normal is about 65%, so she was less than half of normal. She was tolerating the low blood pressure well, with a platelet count of 64, which is pretty low. We normally like to see them above 100. Remember, these people are compromised because they just came out of surgery, so their hematocrit and hemoglobin are normally low, and their platelet counts are normally low, but not less than 100. As a matter of course we give aspirin or enteric-coated aspirin to keep their platelets from aggregating, but for somebody less than 100 we hold that.

I went in and assessed this lady. I was expecting a withered up woman who looked as though she were almost dying, but she actually looked good for 82, although she was a little pale. Her heparin was running and I checked that. She was a small, thin lady. Women with this build frequently have low blood pressure. The woman was in good humor and relatively pain-free. She even joked a bit and carried on a pleasant conversation. It was at the change of shift, so the off-going nurse took the first set of vitals and came to talk to me immediately.

She told me the woman's blood pressure was 78 systolic, and that maybe we should be concerned about that. The off-going nurse did not have report so she didn't know that was normal, and I did. I went in and manually took the patient's blood pressure myself. We also have an Ivac, an automatic blood pressure machine. The machine and I agreed. I got about 82 over 50. So, she was still running pretty low, but not low enough to call the doctor. Her heart rate was 58, which was kind of slow. With the blood pressure being so low, you might expect an increased heart rate, but not so. Her temperature was 97.9, which was pretty normal. Temperatures tend to run cool the first day or so. And her respiratory rate was 20 to 22, somewhere in there, so she was breathing a little bit faster than normal, but not a lot.

I checked her over; she had faint pedal pulses, but they were palpable. In her lungs, she had crackles about halfway up, so her alveoli were popping open. The other part was just straight mucus, which you can hear. So she had lung fields about halfway up, her oxygen saturation was in the low 90s, 92 to 93 on 4 liters of O_2. So she was oxygenating fairly well. We have to remember when we take O_2 sats as opposed to blood gases, it actually measures how many blood cells are not carrying oxygen. So if you have a low hemoglobin and hematocrit and your saturation is high, you may not be carrying a lot of oxygen around because your hemoglobin and hematocrit is low.

Her two chest incisions were in good shape (sometimes there are three if there are chest tubes). I also checked her pacing wires, which normally stay for several days. I checked her ankles, and she had two-plus pitting edema. She was weak, although able to get to the bathroom with assistance; and when I did get her up to go to the bathroom, her blood pressure didn't drop, so it wasn't orthostatic.

I was in a quandary about what to do with this lady, sitting with a blood pressure of 80, and two-plus edema and crackles halfway up her lungs. Sometimes if you don't do anything the crackles may go away, but probably not with that much edema. I couldn't ask for Lasix because of the decreased blood pressure that goes along with it. I thought about some other diuretics, but they pretty much do the same thing—they decrease volume and decrease blood pressure, and her volume was sitting in her tissue instead of her blood vessels. So, she's got heparin running, she's eating and drinking okay. One of the things we can do is exercise the patient, which helps to reduce the edema; the stimulation often helps with the blood pressure. This little lady was only 1 day post-op.

Walking her was tough. She could get to the bathroom okay, but wasn't feeling up to walking the hallways. I was able to get her up and stimulate her somewhat. I got her up in the chair two or three times. She stayed awake, and I made sure she wasn't terribly uncomfortable, with the idea of increasing her blood pressure. I didn't want her to fall asleep because I wanted to get her blood pressure up. But no matter what I did, the blood pressure stayed about 80 or 82. When she was really excited it would scream up to about 88.

I didn't do anything the first day. When I came in the next day, her blood pressure was still about 82 and there was no change in her edema despite her elevated legs. I listened to her lungs and they hadn't changed; there were still scattered crackles throughout the whole bottom half. She was breathing a little more heavily, and her saturation was sitting at around 90. She tolerated it remarkably well; she didn't get dizzy when she stood. She had recovered a bit and was able to move a little better, though she still needed help getting in and out of bed, and getting to the bathroom.

Most people don't have a bowel movement until the third day, and she was no exception. She still had the Foley catheter inserted because of our concern about urine output, which had dropped; she produced only about 120 on day shift. The physician had not come in for rounds, and day shift had not called him about it. He'd say, "What do you want to do—give Lasix and have her blood pressure drop?" So, there we were, the second day, same thing—maybe a little worse, because she was not saturating as well and her lungs were filling up. So what was I going to do?

Now when you give blood, it does increase your vascular pressure, but because of the increased vascular pressure and decreased osmotic pressure, it actually draws fluid out of the vasculature into the tissues. That's why we give Lasix. If we were to give blood, she would probably become more edematous and have more crackles, and fluid in her lungs. I got a chest x-ray, and it showed consolidation in the lower lobes and scattered throughout the upper lobes, meaning there was fluid in the lung.

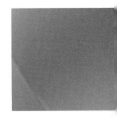

We needed to do something to get that fluid off. I called the physician and said, "What about albumin?" He replied, "Oh, what a good idea." She got one albumin from me. Her blood pressure slowly climbed back up; with the extra osmotic pressure she was able to pull the tissue fluid in. It took about 24 hours, and she went from a two-plus edema to a one-plus. When things started working, they continued to work. We didn't have to give any more albumin; it was enough to push her over the edge. And her activity increased one more day post-op. Her blood pressure soared up into the 90s and she did very well.

THINKING IT THROUGH

1. How did this nurse go about getting needed information? (*Contextual awareness and deciding what to observe and consider*)

2. Can you think of anything you might have done differently? (*Exploring and imagining alternatives*)

3. What else would you have wanted to know in this situation? (*Exploring and imagining alternatives*)

4. How did this nurse validate his assumptions? Were there assumptions he did not validate? (*Assumption recognition and analysis*)

5. In priority order, what would you have done in this situation? (*Reflective skepticism/deciding what to do*)

6. Think of a time when you encountered a patient's response that puzzled you. What did you do? (*Chapter reasoning problem*)

7. Do you think through rationale in the kind of detail used by this nurse? What contributed to his ability to do this? (*Chapter reasoning problem*)

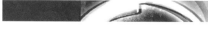

CLINICAL REASONING SKILLS

Comparing Beginners and Experienced Nurses

Think about the beginner scenarios and write down what you think are the key differences between beginners and experienced nurses in relation to:

● Persistence in thinking things through

● Comfort in calling the doctor

● Amount of detail considered in decision making

● Assurance about what to do and ability to provide rationale for actions

● Ability to consider more than one possibility, action, or option

● Ability to think ahead and anticipate what might be problematic for an individual patient

● Ability to prioritize what to do and when to do it

● Skill in seeing what "fits the clinical picture" and what doesn't

● Understanding usual routines, procedures, and patient profiles

● Recognizing how long tasks and patient changes take

List of Scenarios by Clinical Setting and by Beginner Reasoning Problem

Clinical Setting	Scenario Numbers
Medical-Surgical	1, 3, 4, 5, 7, 8, 10, 11, Experienced Nurse Scenario
Maternal-Child	2, 8
Mental Health	6, 9
Community Health	12
Beginner Reasoning Problem	**Scenario Numbers**
Thinking of only one possible explanation	1, 5, 6, 8, 9
Coming up with only one possible action	3, 5, 7, 10, 12
Tending to discount what else is important in the situation	1, 8, 9, 10
Asking others for possibilities, not seeing the options independently	1, 3, 4, 5, 6, 9, 11
Beginning with a routine rather than seeing clinical priorities	1, 7, 10, 11
Missing things during assessments	1, 5, 7, 8, 9, 11
Forgetting to follow up on important details	3, 10
Not thinking ahead about what might happen	2, 3, 6, 10, 11, 12
Not recognizing usual routines, procedures, or patient profiles	3, 6, 11
Not anticipating how long things will take	1, 2, 12

 Ask yourself, "Have I considered all possibilities?"

CHAPTER 5

THE ART OF MAKING ETHICAL DECISIONS

Sound Familiar?

When others' values differ from yours, have you ever:

○ Felt unsure about the right thing to do even though others didn't appear to be bothered by the situation?

○ Wanted to act on a patient's behalf but also wanted to be a loyal employee/student?

○ Been bothered because you noticed patients' needs came second or third behind reimbursement-related or bureaucratic mandates?

○ Recognized that you were the only one who noticed a patient's pain?

○ Believed nothing you could do or say would resolve a difference of opinion between you and other, more experienced professionals?

○ Felt as though patient care had become impersonal, mechanical, or callous, or that no one seemed to assume ongoing responsibility for patient problems or outcomes?

○ Worked with a patient who was different from you and found it difficult to understand their feelings?

○ Felt caught in a tug-of-war of conflicting values or ethical priorities?

○ Disliked a patient or family and had to "make yourself" behave professionally around them?

○ Recalled a situation from the past that continued to bother you because you didn't take the action you felt you should have?

When you don't know what to do, or when you are unsure about something, which of the above behaviors and feelings describe what happens to you?

OBJECTIVES

After completing the learning experiences in this chapter, you will be able to:

- Recognize the influence of the following on ethical decision making: feelings, the environment, and cultural, economic, and gender-based factors.
- Learn to effectively advocate for patients while working in health care delivery systems.
- Develop strategies for dealing with situations that don't seem right.
- Identify approaches you can use when you are unsure of what should be happening in patient care situations.
- Build on previous experience by developing a personal narrative describing a time when you were unsure of your and others' ethical decisions.
- Practice drawing conclusions and supporting arguments for your own ethical decisions.
- Identify ways in which your level of patient involvement affects ethical decision-making.

A Short Scenario

I Can Still Hear Him Screaming

I was on the burn unit doing dressing changes. There was a 4-year-old boy burnt over his trunk and head who was going home that same day. Usually he got morphine sulfate during dressing changes. He had a reputation for screaming during every dressing change, starting with when you walked in the room. Today they didn't want to use morphine because he was going home and the drug requires observation after it is administered. This would have postponed his discharge, which of course would be a problem, because it costs the hospital more money. So they just gave him Tylenol and codeine.

As a student, I had no input about what medications he received. Had I been an RN, I would have refused to help. It took three RNs to hold him down. I felt mean and cruel. We tried distraction and we tried to let him participate in the dressing change. His mom was so upset she couldn't be in the room. He had partial and full-thickness burns over 20% of his body. On that unit, they didn't adjust medications, even the codeine, by body weight or tolerance. I think the nurses were desensitized to the level of pain he was having. It shocked me because I was new to the unit. I think they could have ordered a home health nurse, who could have taught the mother what to watch for with morphine. They should not have kept bringing him back to the hospital every other day for this same routine, and that is what they did. I still remember how he sounded, screaming from the pain.

The conflicting feelings described above reflect many of the ethical dilemmas beginning nurses face. They feel responsible, yet fear they could inflict harm (*Benner, Tanner & Chesla, 1996*). Beginners are not confident enough about how to intervene to make things happen for their patients. Although they would like to persist in making things happen, they also want to please more experienced professionals. Beginning nurses describe situations in which their lack of experience influenced how they felt and acted, when they were not sure the right things were being done; when they felt others were not paying attention to what seemed significant, and when they felt ineffective in advocating for their patients.

When beginners connect emotionally with patients, they may feel especially torn about how to respond to these dilemmas. Often beginners vividly recall details of troubling situations long after they occur, as though they are still unresolved in their mind. Beginners seem to remain stuck in these experiences, replaying them in memory instead of identifying what most affected them about the event and discovering what they may have done to resolve the conflict.

In beginners' stories, troubling events often occurred when others in the situation were distracted, and beginners felt that their patients' needs and their pain weren't being considered. It was often the beginners' emotions that alerted them to the human significance of the situation, yet they felt ineffective in influencing others to resolve the issues.

Ethics researchers indicate that being involved in situations helps people develop an emotional understanding of the most meaningful ethical priorities (*Ben-*

ner, 1989; Gilligan, 1988). Not feeling and not seeing from the patient's perspective tends to create a feeling of distance where caregivers don't really attend to what's right for the patient *(Vetlesen, 1960).* Often in today's health care system, where care is compartmentalized, some professionals don't know their patients as individuals. Today's impersonal health care environment undermines one's sense of responsibility and accountability. It is easier to become disengaged, to make decisions that don't consider patients' values and needs. The antidote to this ethical disengagement or numbing is allowing ourselves to be touched emotionally by our patients *(Benner & Wrubel, 1989).*

In each of the ethical situations described in this chapter, nurses' decisions and actions were based on their ability to feel what the patient was experiencing. Sometimes the ability to understand others' experiences occurred when the nurse and the patient had in common a cultural, economic, religious, geographic, or gender background.

When nurses are aware of their own beliefs and values it can help them understand their patients' views, even when different from their own. In order to be an effective nurse, it is important to connect with patients from a variety of backgrounds.

This chapter is designed to help you become aware of your emotional responses to patient care situations and to discover ways of effectively advocating for patients. As you develop skills in this area, you will become more comfortable dealing with ethical dilemmas.

Recall a Scenario

The scenario described at the beginning of this chapter illustrates a type of ethical dilemma a beginner may experience: a strong sense that something is wrong combined with the need to defer to more experienced professionals. Think back to a time in your clinical practice when you felt uncomfortable about decisions that were being made or actions being taken, but felt powerless to do anything about them.

Write Your Scenario Here

THINKING IT THROUGH

1. What was going on in the situation that bothered you or that didn't seem right? (*Contextual awareness and deciding what to observe and consider*)

2. Which emotional responses influenced how you and others reacted in this situation? (*Contextual awareness and deciding what to observe and consider*)

3. Give one possible explanation for why the beginner was seeing something wrong while others were not. (*Exploring and imagining alternatives*)

4. Which beliefs/values of yours shaped your perceptions and assumptions about this scenario? (*Assumption recognition and analysis*)

5. How could you validate your assumptions? What more would you need to know? (*Assumption recognition and analysis*)

6. What would you have done differently in this situation having had a chance to reflect about it? (*Reflective skepticism/deciding what to do*)

7. In what ways did engagement or involvement influence your beliefs and actions? (*Chapter reasoning problem*)

8. How might you have advocated for this patient? (*Chapter reasoning problem*)

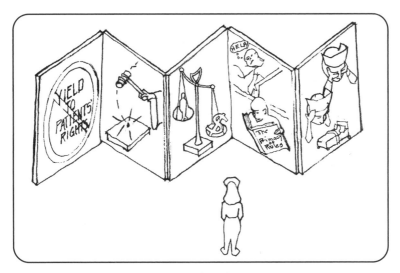

FIGURE 5-1 Ethical dilemmas occur when beginning nurses experience disregard for patients' rights, authoritarian responses, financial concerns taking precedence over patient well-being, health care professionals who don't really "see" the patient, and "following the rules" as driving behaviors.

9. Were you sure the wrong thing was happening? (*Chapter reasoning problem*) (Fig. 5-1)

Ethical Decision Scenarios

Several situations are now presented for you to read. Each scenario is followed by questions to help you reflect about what occurred. As you read through the situations and answer the associated questions, pay attention to the common themes described and compare them to any episodes in which you experienced ethical dilemmas.

Learning or Leering

All the students were in the newborn nursery. It was late in the shift, the census was down, and we were worried about not getting enough babies to do our assessments. One of the nurses on the unit called the nursery to tell us that there was a cleft lip/palate baby coming. The grandparents and the dad were already there. By the

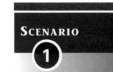

SCENARIO

1

time the baby arrived, the doctors had determined she had a brain stem and nothing else. There was only one nostril. She was having seizures. I tried to step back because the father was young and this was a devastating experience for him.

Unfortunately, not all of the other students stepped back. One was holding a healthy baby, peering at the one with the defect. "I don't think the nurses would want you to stand up and feed this baby," I said. "Why don't you sit down?" My voice was stern. The student pulled her rocker near the new baby and continued feeding the other child. Seeing the normal baby had to be hard for the family. All the other students were lined up staring too. I kept thinking, "This family has waited 9 months for this child and they love it." Many students came from other units to see the baby; they were just standing there gawking.

I was bothered, so I decided to tell our instructor. I said, "We need to talk about our boundaries in conference; about when to step back." We never did talk in conference, although the instructor talked to individual students. This was a new life, and the family probably had so many expectations for the baby. People were lining the viewing window. The father was looking at everyone as they looked on. There was a look of embarrassment on his face. The mother was still in the recovery room and only the dad and the grandparents were there. We're supposed to be patient advocates, concerned about the family. I'm not sure, but I think because I am a recent mom, I could feel more of what the family was feeling.

I'm not sure why, but the following week, when the family could have taken the baby home, they refused. The baby lived 3 weeks. They were withholding feedings, but the baby was transferred to a larger hospital where they started feedings. I don't know if I understand why they would feed a child without a brain. Maybe for organ transplants and harvesting or so the baby wouldn't have a painful death. It turned out to be only the 12th baby anywhere born with that particular anomaly. The head was really large and the face was round. There hadn't been any signs that the baby would be born like this. The mom's drug screen and history had been negative. The baby didn't cry. The sound she made was not normal. I can still hear her. The neonatologist was just out of school and asked another doctor to talk to the family.

The atmosphere of modern technology and large hospitals, where there are many people in and out of the room, makes us all a bit callous. We are required to ask questions to complete our write-ups; there is very little time, and we want to obtain all the data and experience we can before we graduate. We need experience, but are supposed to be compassionate too. When we just pop into the situation for a day of clinical, we don't plug into the feelings and the people; the goal takes over. But we need to remember, patients matter too.

THINKING IT THROUGH

Below are questions to guide your reflective thinking about the above scenario. We have included answers as examples of appropriate responses. Please keep in mind that there may be other responses that are also correct. The important thing is for you to think about the scenario and generate as many responses as possible.

You may find it useful to try to answer the questions yourself before looking at the suggested answers.

1. What factors influenced the "peering" students' behaviors in this situation? (*Contextual awareness and deciding what to observe and consider*)
   - Not being involved with the family; no (or very limited) awareness of family
   - Not imagining the situation from the family's perspective
   - Not having enough patients and feeling a need to "get the paper work done"
   - Curiosity about something very unusual/never seen before

2. What is one thing you might have done in this situation to make the outcome better? (*Exploring and imagining alternatives*)
   - Done something to increase others' awareness of the family and their feelings, such as asking the group of students to meet with you in a room away from the nursery and describing what you knew or were feeling about the family and how they might have been feeling
   - Asked the group how they would feel if this were their baby
   - Spoken to the charge nurse to seek her input about the situation

3. Are there other resources that needed to be mobilized? (*Exploring and imagining alternatives*)
   - Nurses who knew the family might have describe what they were experiencing
   - If the hospital had a social worker or a mental health clinical nurse specialist, they could have been contacted.

4. What was taken for granted in this situation? (*Assumption recognition and analysis*)
   - The family wouldn't care if they were observed.
   - It was OK for professionals who are learning to look at the baby.
   - The family was influenced not to take the baby home by others' responses.

5. Which belief/values were most important to consider in this situation? (*Assumption recognition and analysis*)
   - The family's feelings were more important than the students' curiosity or learning.
   - It was important to help the family with their reactions to this baby, and the presence of students watching everything significantly interfered with this.

6. Why was it important to intervene in this situation? (*Reflective skepticism/ deciding what to do*)
   - The students were new and didn't yet have an awareness of others in the situation. Helping them see how others were experiencing the situation might have helped them in the future. The family might have been influenced by others' reactions.

7. What rationale did the student have for her decisions and comments? (*Reflective skepticism/deciding what to do*)
   - She imagined what it might feel like to have people looking at her child as if it were a "freak."

- She identified that being busy and rushed in clinical can influence students.

8. Have you ever experienced feeling like you could still hear a child cry, or remember the look on someone's face even after the event was over? Describe the situation if you have experienced a similar feeling (*Chapter reasoning problem*)

    - I remember I came onto a unit. All the nurses were sitting around charting, talking to each other, waiting for report, and hearing this very old patient cry out, "Help me! Help me! Help me!" No one seemed to even hear her or care about her pleas. I was new to the unit and was afraid to go into the patient's room to check on her. I mean, no one was getting up to go to her room. What would they think if I did? I didn't even know where things were. Later, I was assigned to that patient. The poor lady was in terrible pain, but the staff didn't want to give her anything for it. She moaned and cried out all morning. I felt so helpless. I can still see her. I still feel very bad about that day. It just was very wrong. I should have done something, but I didn't.

9. What did the student mean when she commented, "You don't plug into the feelings and the people; the goal takes over when you pop into a situation for a day"? (*Chapter reasoning problem*)

    - She probably meant that when students come to clinical experiences once per week or just rotate through a particular clinical unit, they don't get to know patients or get involved in personal meanings of situations. When people are not involved, or don't know anything about the people in a situation, it's easy to discount their feelings and the meanings of the situation to the people.

10. This beginner felt that others were not attending to the needs of the father. What could she have done to help people see the father's discomfort? (*Chapter reasoning problem*)

    - She could have shared her perceptions with the students.
    - She could have asked them to think about how they would feel in a similar situation.

SCENARIO 2

I Wish I Had Let Her Family Stay

I was working on a medical tele floor with two RNs and three LVNs, each with 8 to 10 patients. An LVN had called in sick, and they weren't able to cover her shift. In report I had one cancer patient with a morphine drip. Her roommate was an East Indian woman admitted for liver problems. Her daughter repeatedly asked to stay the night. Our policy is that this is not done unless a patient is critical or terminal. We've had some gang problems recently. We were busy so we didn't talk about it much—the charge nurse just went in and told her, "No," pretty quickly.

In the next room was a man with a GI bleed, incontinent, with a guaiac-positive stool. Next to him was a stroke patient who was confused and yelling at staff. I did rounds to make sure the IVs were in place. I found the man with a GI bleed crawling out through the bed rails. I gave him the urinal after repositioning him. I did my midnight medications. The stroke patient was trying to get out of bed, so I put a Posey on him after changing his bed. At 2:30, the cancer patient got an IV medication. While I was giving it, I glanced at her roommate and noticed shadows on her face. I went over there and blood was all over her face. I asked the supervisor about whether to code her and she said we legally had to. There was so much blood. We had to suction her first. The MD from ER came in and we called the code. We closed the curtains but we could not clean her up because in our hospital every death is a coroner's case. We couldn't even remove the IVs.

The MD telephoned and the entire East Indian family arrived to start their mourning pattern. We got the daughter a chair; she couldn't even stand up seeing her mother covered with blood. The charge nurse was mortified because she hadn't let the daughter stay the night. We rationalized that it was better the daughter had not seen everything. I suppose it was esophageal varices bleeding out through her mouth and nose. They can happen so fast. I will never forget that night. There was no ascites or anything except a history of liver disease to alert me to pay more attention to her. If I had the night to live over, I would have talked to the daughter and gotten a feel for what made her want to spend the night before we just said, "No" automatically.

THINKING IT THROUGH

1. What was going on in the context that influenced what happened in this situation? (*Contextual awareness and deciding what to observe and consider*)

2. What emotional responses influenced how the beginner reacted in this situation? (*Contextual awareness and deciding what to observe and consider*)

3. Which assumptions did not make sense in this situation? (*Assumption recognition and analysis*)

4. What priorities were missed? (*Reflective skepticism/deciding what to do*)

5. What was done? Why was it done? (*Reflective skepticism/deciding what to do*)

6. What bothered the beginner most about this situation? (*Chapter reasoning problem*)

7. Describe how the beginner's sense of involvement changed as this situation unfolded. (*Chapter reasoning problem*)

8. What difference did it make in this situation that the woman who died was East Indian? (*Chapter reasoning problem*)

9. Assume that you felt it would be all right to let the family stay. What could you have said to the charge nurse? (*Chapter reasoning problem*)

SCENARIO

3

When Does the Patient Come First?

I was watching a central line being inserted. They were trying to place the patient into a Trendelenburg position to get the vein engorged so they would avoid nicking the lung. The patient had been involved in a gang fight. He had an abdominal stab wound that had severed his superior mesenteric artery, which resulted in ischemia and death of most of his ileum. The bedside doctors told the patient that he had the bare minimum of his ileum to survive. The central catheter would be inserted to supply the patient with TPN (total parenteral nutrition) while the anastomosed ends of the intestine healed. The patient was a young African-American, in his early 20s, who appeared to be a bit overwhelmed by what happened to him. He had to have the reasons for the procedure explained a couple of times before he signed the consent.

The beds on the unit won't rise to the up position and the Trendelenburg at the same time, so the doctors decided to put pillows under the patient's legs and buttocks to achieve Trendelenburg. A resident and two doctors were in the room to perform the procedure. The patient began to shiver, so I put another blanket on him, thinking he was cold. I said, "You look cold." He responded, "I'm not cold, my stomach is killing me." It took me a minute to realize that the patient was not shivering because he was cold, but because of how he was positioned. He was supporting his back with his abdominal muscles. He complained to the doctors that his back was killing him. They told him to just lie still, they would be done in 15 minutes. I told the patient, "I'll be right back with some towels to support your back."

When I got back, the doctors had established a sterile field from the patient's head to his knees and were starting the procedure. They said they didn't want to disturb the field. I lost interest in watching the procedure because the patient looked so miserable. I had to leave the room. I couldn't watch him being so uncomfortable just for the sake of the cost involved in setting up a new sterile field. I felt the doctors discounted the patient and me as well. In the last year, I have wondered about myself and whether I was more interested in diagnoses and the medical aspects of nursing education or caring for patients. This scenario answered that question for me: I was more interested in the comfort of the patient than the procedure.

THINKING IT THROUGH

1. What emotional responses influenced how the beginner reacted to this situation? (*Contextual awareness and deciding what to observe and consider*)

2. What were some of the factors that influenced the way the doctors were behaving in this situation? (*Contextual awareness and deciding what to observe and consider; chapter reasoning problem*)

3. Describe one thing the beginner could have done in this situation. (*Exploring and imagining alternatives*)

4. What were the doctors taking for granted? What was the beginner taking for granted? (*Assumption recognition and analysis*)

5. In what way did beliefs/values shape assumptions in this situation? (*Assumption recognition and analysis*)

6. Why was it important to intervene in this situation? (*Reflective skepticism/ deciding what to do*)

7. Do you think the doctors were at all engaged with the patient as a person? If they were engaged, how do you think this might have influenced their reactions to the patient? (*Chapter reasoning problem*)

8. What could the beginner have said to the physicians to help them acknowledge the patient's pain? (*Chapter reasoning problem*)

9. Have you ever experienced a situation where cultural or socioeconomic factors made a difference? If so, describe that scenario. (*Chapter reasoning problem*)

10. The beginner was so uncomfortable about what was happening that he left the room. Why didn't he advocate for the patient's comfort? Think of a time when this happened to you. As you think of it now, how could you been more of an advocate? (*Chapter reasoning problem*)

I Can't Believe She Hit Him

I was working graveyard shift on weekends. It was an Alzheimer's unit. One man needed his Depends changed and he was angry, flailing and kicking. He hit the other aide I was working with on the chin. I thought people went into this field because they wanted to help others. She hit him back with her fist. She was yelling and telling me to hold his arms. I asked her to be gentle. She hog-tied him and slapped him repeatedly on the bottom. I told her I would not help her anymore. I went to call the charge nurse. She said the other aide was having a bad night and I was overreacting. I could see fear in other patients' eyes when this aide woke them up. She had no compassion. I decided I would tell the nursing supervisor. She told me she would deal with it. At the same time, she told me they had trouble getting staff. I thought about sending a note to the family, but I decided not to. I let the other nurses know to watch out for this aide. I witnessed a few other incidents and then I decided to quit. I often wonder what would have happened if I had called Adult Protective Services. It took a lot of energy to work in an extended care facility. I always came home exhausted. I had to learn to walk out of the room sometimes. I said to myself over and over, "What would I do if this were my mom or dad?"

THINKING IT THROUGH

1. What factors influenced the beginner's behavior in this situation? (*Contextual awareness and deciding what to observe and consider*)

2. What else would you want to know in this situation? (*Exploring and imagining alternatives*)

3. Imagine a different way of reacting to this incident. What would be the likely result of this action? (*Exploring and imagining alternatives*)

4. What were some of the beginner's assumptions in this situation? What assumptions could you add? (*Assumption recognition and analysis*)

5. How could you validate your assumptions with the aide? (*Assumption recognition and analysis*)

6. Why was it important to intervene in this situation? (*Reflective skepticism/deciding what to do*)

7. What is one thing you could have done to help the aide see how this behavior affected the patient? (*Chapter reasoning problem*)

8. If you were a licensed nurse in this situation, what would you have been required to do by law in response to what you observed? (*Chapter reasoning problem*)

9. If the employer decided to influence the aide's job standing, how might the "whistle-blowing" statutes protect her? (*Chapter reasoning problem*)

10. In your area, how would you contact Adult Protective Services if your employer declined to do this when abuse was reported? (*Chapter reasoning problem*)

11. This beginner felt a great sense of responsibility but nonetheless did not persist in advocating for the patient. Think of a time when you did not persist in advocating for a patient. Now how would you respond to that situation? (*Chapter reasoning problem*)

The System Tied My Hands

SCENARIO
5

I was working as a consultant to a rural convalescent home, doing nutritional assessments one day a week. It was a quality assurance type of thing. This woman was a 350 pound, new admit, 5 feet 6 inches tall. She was 60 years old and on Lasix. My main concern was that she was on a 900-calorie liquid diet for weight loss with open lesions on her legs. She was almost bedridden, but she got up to use the bedside commode. Her albumin was low; she had pitting edema, which could have been from the low protein diet. She had no roommate, and her family never visited. The nurses avoided this patient because they said she was a bit manipulative. I never did ask what they meant by that. The patient told me the doctor had talked her into losing weight. I told her it was also important to work on wound healing, since she had gaping sores. I talked about how raising her metabolism by raising her mobility would be good. I realized she was lonely and depressed so she had trouble making herself get out of the room. I calculated she needed 2,000 to 2,500 calories minimum for wound healing with 80 grams of protein in comparison to the 40 grams she was getting.

I talked with the RNs, who said there was nothing they could do because all other nursing homes in the area had refused to take her. I called the doctor but couldn't reach him, and he didn't call back. One week later I spoke with the administrator and the director of nursing. The doctor was a thin 60-year-old man who put everyone in the facility on a 2-gram low-sodium diet. He had a reputation for being a fanatic about weight loss. Finally I got to talk to him, but he said he didn't think it was important to consider the amount of protein in a diet. He didn't care that 1000 calories wouldn't support her wound healing. He was the medical director; so I couldn't go over his authority. He was the top authority. By this time the patient was no longer feisty. She still had edema, but he discontinued the Lasix because she was in renal failure. The state was scheduled to arrive one week later for an inspection. I could not chart that I agreed with the doctor. The patient started drinking a nutritional supplement (Ensure). Now she had stage 2 decubitus ulcers and had to be lifted by four nurses. I talked to the state inspector. The state said they knew of the doctor's reputation, but it was a problem because in that rural area no other doctors wanted the medical director's job. Finally the patient got transferred to an acute care facility. The situation has always stuck in my mind. I quit that company, but I ran into the dietitian for that facility a few months later at a conference, and she mentioned how bad the doctor was too. Maybe I should have called the patient's daughter, but the nurses told me she didn't care. Maybe I should have talked more to the patient about her right to refuse the doctor's order. Patients don't always understand that they have rights.

THINKING IT THROUGH

1. What things were happening simultaneously that affected the beginner in this situation? (*Contextual awareness and deciding what to observe and consider*)

2. What else would you have wanted to know? (*Contextual awareness and deciding what to observe and consider*)

3. What is one thing you would have wanted to do? (*Exploring and imagining alternatives*)

4. What are two additional possibilities? (*Exploring and imagining alternatives*)

5. What was taken for granted in this situation? (*Assumption recognition and analysis*)

6. What beliefs/values shaped assumptions in this situation? (*Assumption recognition and analysis*)

7. Why was it important to intervene in this situation? (*Reflective skepticism/ deciding what to do*)

8. Contrast the beginner's and the doctor's sense of connection with the patient. (*Chapter reasoning problem*)

9. What difference did it make in this situation that the convalescent hospital was in a rural area? What difference did it make that the woman was overweight? (*Chapter reasoning problem*)

10. This beginner thought of two ways of advocating for the patient in this situation. What were they? Which of these would you have done? (*Chapter reasoning problem*)

I Can't Believe He Said That!

I was working with a 27-year-old woman who was admitted to the hospital with a premature rupture of membrane and meconium-stained amniotic fluid. She was started on ampicillin. For the next 22 hours, she experienced mild sporadic contractions, and the baby showed no signs of distress. Pitocin was started, and during the early stages of labor her blood pressure started to climb to 154/90. Her platelets were dropping, she had HELLP syndrome, and urine dips were positive for trace amounts of protein. Because of this, magnesium sulfate was begun. Her grandmother, boyfriend, aunt, and cousin were taking turns coaching her labor. I was at the foot of the bed supporting her left leg. The doctor was positioned at the foot of the bed applying perineal massage.

As the time of delivery approached, I asked her boyfriend if he would like to move to the foot of the bed and watch the baby as it was delivered. We were all exhausted, and finally the big moment was about to happen. We'd all been through Lamaze together and assisted the mother through this difficult labor. I thought it was the least I could do. As we prepared to switch places, the doctor snapped, "You stay right there." Glaring at me, the doctor ordered the boyfriend to return to the head of the bed. We were all shocked at this outburst and obeyed her command. After the delivery of a healthy 8-pound baby boy, the boyfriend expressed his disappointment to the doctor about not being able to view the birth. The doctor didn't really answer him. She just walked out the door. What could I have said to the doctor that would have helped?

THINKING IT THROUGH

1. What influenced the boyfriend's and nurse's behaviors in this delivery situation? (*Contextual awareness and deciding what to observe and consider*)

2. What is one possible explanation for the doctor's behavior? (*Exploring and imagining alternatives*)

3. What was taken for granted in this situation? (*Assumption recognition and analysis*)

4. What values shaped these assumptions? (*Assumption recognition and analysis*)

5. What would you have done differently after reflecting about this situation? (*Reflective skepticism/deciding what to do*)

6. Why was it important to intervene in this situation? (*Reflective skepticism/deciding what to do*)

7. What could you have said to the doctor to help her understand the boyfriend's desire to see the birth? (*Chapter reasoning problem*)

8. This beginner did not advocate for the boyfriend. Would you have felt the same way? Describe how you would have felt. How do you imagine the boyfriend felt? (*Chapter reasoning problem*)

SCENARIO 7

Does the Order Always Come First?

I was working on a subacute unit with a new admit patient who was unsteady on her feet and needed assistance to the bathroom. She was mostly nonverbal and had her teeth clenched stoically. She had been crying and telling her son she had been raped. He acted as though he believed her. After I set up her food tray, she just fell into the food and stayed there. I helped her sit up, wiped away the food, and then I fed her because she would not eat on her own. She did not interact with me at all. Later the LVN asked for my assistance to hold this patient so she could insert a catheter, which the doctor had ordered to obtain a urine specimen. I questioned the reasoning, pointing out that it may be traumatic to her if she was indeed raped. The LVN said, "The doctor ordered it and we are going to do it."

We walked into the room and quickly told the patient what we were going to do and then began to clean the patient for catheter insertion. The patient immediately began to kick and scream. When the LVN tried to explain things again, she closed her eyes and her mouth and turned her head away. We tried to do it as quickly as possible and had to ask a third person to help us hold the patient down.

I felt very uneasy about this situation. I would have liked to know her psychiatric history, why the catheter had been ordered for a urine specimen, and if it was important enough to traumatize the patient as we obviously did. I was uncomfortable not knowing whether the patient had the right to refuse the treatment. Although she did not say in words, "I refuse to have this done," her behavior and screaming showed that she was refusing. She was not on conservatorship or a legal hold. When something like this happens, my frustration is from having to continue on to the next patient, and hurry to catch up with my work. I have to rush home, get a little sleep and go on to the next day's challenges, whatever they happen to be. I feel that my schedule is so disjointed that I can never really finish anything completely, such as asking about the rationale for her catheterization. It just takes too much time, which is something I don't have right now. It seems all of health care is too pushed, too rushed nowadays.

THINKING IT THROUGH

1. What factors influenced this beginner's behavior? (*Contextual awareness and deciding what to observe and consider*)

2. What was important about this situation and what was not important? (*Contextual awareness and deciding what to observe and consider*)

3. What is one thing you could have done in this situation? (*Exploring and imagining alternatives*)

4. What was taken for granted in this situation? (*Assumption recognition and analysis*)

5. What assumptions about time and patient's rights influenced decisions in this situation? (*Assumption recognition and analysis*)

6. Why was it important to intervene in this situation? (*Reflective skepticism/ deciding what to do*)

7. What kept this beginner from being more assertive in this situation? (*Chapter reasoning problem*)

8. What would have bothered you most in this situation? (*Chapter reasoning problem*)

9. Have you ever gone home from clinical or work and had "ethical issues" remain on your mind? (*Chapter reasoning problem*)

10. What could this beginning nurse have done to get the other nurse to place herself in the patient's situation? If you're sure something is not being done right, how can you make yourself persist? What if you're not sure? (*Chapter reasoning problem*)

Neither My Patient Nor I Matter

After SICU report, the charge nurse briefly introduced me to my preceptor for the day. She looked at me and then looked away, with an expression that suggested she was thinking, "Oh, great, another new graduate." When I smiled at her and received no response in return I knew it was going to be a tough day. My preceptor took off down the hall to receive report on one of her patients. While she was doing this, I went to see my patient. He was looking at me in distress. His alarms were going off, and I could tell he needed suctioning. I was surprised that no one responded to his respiratory alarms. So I bravely approached my preceptor who was speaking to another nurse. I was ignored like I didn't exist. I felt so small. But I proceeded to tell the nurse about my patient's alarms. The other nurse who was speaking to my preceptor stated in a short voice, "We'll be there when we're done!" I could not accept this response so I said, "But I think he really needs to be suctioned and his alarms won't stop." The nurse just said, "We'll be there shortly." They didn't say how long or anything. She wasn't even looking at me as she said this. I was worried about my patient, so I went to the night nurse who had cared for him during the night shift and was ready to leave. I said, "Can you please help me? My patient's respiratory alarms are going off and I think he needs suctioning." She just said to me, "You need to go to your nurse." I told her I had, and she responded with the same answer. At this point I was ready to cry. I felt helpless and no one would listen to me. The last thing I wanted was to go up to my preceptor again and be treated like nothing. One more rejection was either going to make me blow up or break down. Fortunately, I calmed my feelings and went back to talk to my preceptor.

THINKING IT THROUGH

1. What things were happening simultaneously in this situation that affected this beginner? (*Contextual awareness and deciding what to observe and consider*)

2. What emotional responses influenced how the beginner was reacting in this situation? (*Contextual awareness and deciding what to observe and consider*)

3. What about this situation have you seen before, and what is different? (*Contextual awareness and deciding what to observe and consider*)

4. What is one possible explanation for why the preceptor was not responding to the beginner's request for help? (*Exploring and imagining alternatives*)

5. What other resources might the beginner have mobilized? (*Exploring and imagining alternatives*)

6. What was taken for granted in this situation? (*Assumption recognition and analysis*)

7. Which beliefs/values shaped assumptions in this situation? (*Assumption recognition and analysis*)

8. What would you have done differently after reflecting about this situation? (*Reflective skepticism/deciding what to do*)

9. What might have improved the involvement the beginner had with the preceptor? (*Chapter reasoning problem*)

10. This beginner was desperate for help, but even more desperate not to be poorly treated or to feel dumb. Think of a time when you felt like this beginner—afraid to persist. Imagine yourself feeling very sure of what needed to be done. What would you say? (*Chapter reasoning problem*)

Being Bounced Around

SCENARIO 9

I had a 68-year-old Hispanic female patient who was seen for treatment of chronic back and neck pain. She had been dealing with chronic pain for 30 years. She recently increased her prescription of Vicodin from 2 q.d. to 3 q.d. when she started a new volunteer job. The resident assigned to evaluate her was stern and impatient with her. She tried to remain positive during the evaluation, but she almost started crying on three occasions. She was frustrated and felt bounced around, as though people were not taking her pain seriously. Her last doctor insinuated that she was seeking treatment only to obtain Vicodin.

While the resident stepped out to consult with his attending physician regarding a treatment plan, I sat to talk with the patient for about 20 minutes. I then went out to get her some water and overheard the resident saying, "She'll think I'm the best doctor in the world if I give her a Vicodin prescription." He was laughing. I had an overwhelming urge to say something in the patient's defense. I said, "I don't believe drug abuse is the issue with her. She told me she is open to any pain treatment including physical therapy. She is just tired of being bounced from one doctor to another." Neither one of the doctors looked at me when I spoke. I felt they weren't really listening to me. I felt as though I hadn't done any good. Later I heard the doctors had decided on an aggressive pain control plan, including a Vicodin prescription and a TENS unit.

THINKING IT THROUGH

1. What about this situation have you seen before? (*Contextual awareness and deciding what to observe and consider*)

2. What emotions influenced how the beginner responded to this situation? (*Contextual awareness and deciding what to observe and consider*)

3. What is one possible explanation for the resident's response to this patient? (*Exploring and imagining alternatives*)

4. Which beliefs/values shaped assumptions in this situation? (*Assumption recognition and analysis*)

5. What would you have done differently in this situation? (*Reflective skepticism/deciding what to do*)

6. How might the resident's response have differed if he had spent more time talking to the patient to find out about her pain experiences? (*Chapter reasoning problem*)

7. What might you have said to the physician to help him better understand this patient's experience? (*Chapter reasoning problem*)

8. The beginner felt ignored, but later discovered that the doctors acted on something she had said. Think of a situation where you felt sure of what you were saying, but someone seemed to ignore what you were saying. How did you advocate for your point of view? How has that been different in situations when you were not sure of yourself? (*Chapter reasoning problem*)

9. In what way did gender or cultural influences affect this situation? (*Chapter reasoning problem*)

10. How would you have approached the patient? What would you have said? (*Chapter reasoning problem*)

Discharge Him, Suicidal or Not

SCENARIO
10

A 35-year-old man was admitted to the inpatient unit of a mental health hospital owned by the company he worked for as a physician's assistant. He had lost 10 pounds within a few weeks after finding out his wife wanted a divorce after 17 years. She had been involved in an affair with another man, which his 16-year-old daughter knew about but had not told him. The wife had been in contact with her high school sweetheart over the last 2 years and had been spending family money to travel to Los Angeles to visit the boyfriend, saying she was going there to maintain her business contacts in the area. The patient had been sleeping only 2 to 3 hours per night, even with 100 milligrams of Benadryl. He had taken some Prozac from the free medication supplies at work, hoping to treat his depression, but began to feel suicidal and voluntarily admitted himself. He had planned to suffocate or shoot himself (there were guns in the home).

Documentation in the chart indicated that he would be placed on a mandatory psychiatric hold if he tried to leave while he was still feeling suicidal. He had a history of obsessive compulsive disorder as a child and a need to be perfect and in control. He was very concerned about confidentiality, because he worked for another branch of the same hospital and did not want his employer to know about his admission. He was admitted on a Saturday and provided the hospital with his insurance information and his wife's insurance card, although he hoped they would not utilize her insurance. He did not want his wife to know he had been hospitalized. Finances were difficult, and he was facing a divorce.

On Monday, he found out that his insurance did not provide for inpatient care although the hospital had assured him it would when he was admitted because "Blue Shield policies always do." When the physician heard that pre-authorization had not been received and that no other insurance was available, he said, "Discharge him, suicidal or not."

The nurses were told to get the patient's signature on a form that stated he was responsible for paying the $3000 bill himself. I was also told to elicit his cooperation. With the help of another nurse, we encouraged the patient to identify feelings and questions regarding the insurance issue and then contacted the hospital administrator. After talking to the patient, the administrator admitted the hospital had made a mistake by not following its standard insurance-verification procedures during a weekend. The patient was discharged after talking to the administrator, but declined to sign a form saying he was responsible for the bill. He left the hospital with a crisis line contact and list of outpatient therapists. He continued to question whether or not he would be billed for the 2½ days of services he received, but was not given a clear answer.

I was reassured that the patient had not signed the form and that the administrator had admitted the hospital was at fault. I felt I had witnessed an example of why there is a need for greater patient advocacy. I was troubled that the patient was being discharged with worries beyond those he had when admitted for suicidal ideation.

THINKING IT THROUGH

1. What was happening just before this incident that made a difference? (*Contextual awareness and deciding what to observe and consider*)

2. Why were the staff and administrator interested in discharging this patient? (*Exploring and imagining alternatives*)

3. Were there others who might have helped develop more alternatives? (*Exploring and imagining alternatives*)

4. Which assumptions contributed to the problem in this situation? (*Assumption recognition and analysis*)

5. What else might have worked in this situation? (*Reflective skepticism/deciding what to do*)

6. Which aspects of this situation were most troubling to this beginner? (*Chapter reasoning problem*)

7. Which aspects would have bothered you most? (*Chapter reasoning problem*)

8. This beginner felt a strong sense of responsibility for the patient. She also felt the patient's needs were not being recognized. How could she have influenced the administrator's decision? (*Chapter reasoning problem*)

What to Do About Tom

I had been working daily for 4 days, and in report I had become familiar with a patient named Tom who had been admitted 5 days earlier. Tom was well known to the staff because he had owned an ambulance service in town and was one of the local EMTs . However, at 74 years old, with a 140-pack-a-year history of smoking Camel no-filters, and supposedly drinking 1 to 1½ fifths of whiskey daily, Tom's body was giving out and he was hospitalized for chest pains and shortness of breath.

Tom knew the progression of illnesses such as his because he had defibrillated heart attack victims in his ambulance, had intubated COPD patients who had stopped breathing, and had seen bloody froth come from between the lips of people in severe congestive heart failure. His current diagnosis was exacerbation of COPD, rule out MI, and uncontrolled hypertension. In addition, he had inoperable CAD with a left ventricular ejection fraction of less than 25%. Each day in report, the night staff would tell how they caught Tom smoking in the bathroom, or how he had nearly coded when he got out of bed to smoke in the bathroom.

Despite his intimate knowledge of his condition, Tom refused to be comply with his doctor's recommendations to quit smoking and drinking and to change his diet. Today was my first day working with Tom, and the LVN told me to expect to meet the crustiest, most ornery person I would ever encounter. I decided to assess Tom as the last of my six patients because I knew from report that he was stable, a DNR patient, and probably a time-consuming patient.

I entered Tom's room at about 8:30 and he looked dusky. He was sitting on the toilet complaining of chest pains. I immediately helped him back to bed. His vital signs were T = 99.5, R = 28, BP = 210/120, and O_2 sat 92% on 5 liters of O_2 via cannula. He had widespread expiratory wheezes and bilateral rales, strong peripheral pulses, peripheral edema, and complaints of chest pain. I gave his morning medications of nitropaste, 240 mg Cardizem, 80 mg IV push Lasix, 80 mg IV push methylprednisolone, slo mag, K Dur, and a prn of 1.25 mg IV push Vasotec for SBP greater than 180. Tom told me he realized each day could be his last, and he just wanted to enjoy himself for as long as possible.

Later that day his 34-year-old wife came in and wheeled him out to the parking lot, where they smoked a few cigarettes. Tom asked me to open his lunch over the table bed, where he had a salt shaker hidden. He started salting his food, but of course was on a 2 gram sodium diet. As he shook that salt shaker, he told me he was a desert rat from way back and he had to have his salt. I told him I should take his tray away and bring him one without salt. He looked at me like he would like to kill me. It was a man-to-man sort of look. I thought about taking the salt shaker and about the stress of searching his room after each visitor. I had a duty to the hospital to get Tom back home before his DRGs ran out and the hospital had to "eat" the cost of his treatment. I decided to let him decide about his life. He was well educated, alert, oriented, and a strong-willed man.

He nearly coded at least two more times during his hospital stay, and then was discharged home 8 days later. But all in all, I think it was better for him to decide whether or not to be compliant with his treatment and I would probably make the same decision again today. He chose to live in a mountain community where personal autonomy was important, and he was clear about the life choices he was making.

Removing his chance to make a choice somehow seemed worse for him, but it was hard for me to decide whether to advocate for what was best for the patient's health, the hospital, or the patient's decisions.

THINKING IT THROUGH

1. What factors influenced the behavior of the beginner in this situation? (*Contextual awareness and deciding what to observe and consider*)

2. What about this situation have you seen before and what is new? (*Contextual awareness and deciding what to observe and consider*)

3. What else would you have wanted to know in this situation? (*Exploring and imagining alternatives*)

4. Which beliefs/values were most important to the beginner in this situation? (*Assumption recognition and analysis*)

5. What else might have worked in this situation? (*Reflective skepticism/deciding what to do*)

6. Having decided what was wrong/happening in this situation, what would have been the best response? (*Reflective skepticism/deciding what to do*)

7. How did the beginner's knowledge of Tom as a person influence his response? (*Chapter reasoning problem*)

8. Would any aspect of this situation have troubled you? Please explain your answer. (*Chapter reasoning problem*)

9. What geographic and gender-based influences made a difference in this situation? (*Chapter reasoning problem*)

10. This beginner involved himself enough with the patient to understand his behavior. What influence did this knowledge have on the beginner's decision not to persist in changing Tom's behaviors? What do you think the nurse's response would have been if he didn't know him as well? (*Chapter reasoning problem*)

In a Nutshell

It is important for beginners to be aware of the potential for being so focused on a skill or a small part of a situation that the larger context is not recognized or experienced. This can lead to decisions that don't consider what's right and what's important to those who are involved in the situation. It is also true that the beginner can sometimes be more involved than more experienced professionals, partly because of the newness of a situation. It can be very intimidating when others are not acknowledging or responding to a patient's needs in a way that you would want them to, or when you are not feeling that you can assert your opinions or advocate strongly enough for the patient. As you define your role with others and as your confidence in your perceptions and decisions increases, you will improve your ability to be assertive and to help others become engaged with patients' needs.

THINKING IT THROUGH

1. Recall a situation in which you had to make a decision and you knew little about the people involved in the situation. Compare that to a situation in which you knew a great deal about the people. What were the differences in the decision making? Look again at all of the clinical scenarios and see if being involved with others influenced the professionals' level of engagement and focus on the patients' needs.

2. List elements in the chapter scenarios described by beginners as contributing to or preceding the episodes of ethical dilemmas or decision-making.

3. In what ways did the beginners cope with the differences between their values and others' values and/or behaviors?

4. In each of the situations, contrast the beginner's involvement with the patient compared to that of the other professionals in the situation.

5. What might the beginners have done in these scenarios to increase the involvement of the staff with the patient? How do you imagine that would have changed decisions?

6. What can you do when you have a different assessment of decisions than others because of what you know about a patient? What are some assertive behaviors you could try? Think of one assertive activity that you would have been willing to use if you had been the beginner in each of the scenarios presented.

7. Review scenarios 2, 3, 4, 6, and 10. Identify the cultural, economic, religious, gender-based, and geographic factors that influenced the situations. Which of these scenarios would have been most difficult for you to deal with and why?

Create Your Mind Map*

Step #1

Identify the central themes that describe the beginner's reactions and feelings in the chapter scenarios. Place the feelings in the center of the page, and draw a large circle around them. *Hint: Review scenarios and answers to the questions in the "In a Nutshell" section.*

Step #2

Think of factors that contributed to these feelings and reactions. Draw a circle around each one and place them around the large circle in the center of the page.

Step #3

Identify approaches you would use to cope with these ethical issues. Write down the key words and place them in a box. Draw a line from the box to the appropriate circle.

Step #4

You may also use pictures to portray the central coping theme. Mind map subtopics may include:

- How beginners cope with value discrepancies
- Situational factors that contributed to value differences among the beginner and other professional staff members
- Emotions that influenced feelings and actions
- Suggestions for helping people get involved in the situation
- Ways to respond when there are value discrepancies
- Strategies for persisting in making things happen/advocating for patients

---

*For Steps 1 to 3, use a separate sheet of paper if necessary.

Place Your Mind Map Here

Let's See Another Scenario

Review the approaches outlined in this chapter and in your mind map for responding to situations in which you disagree with what is taking place. Select an approach that suits you and describe a scenario where you tried or thought about trying this approach. Describe what you did, what worked, and what you would have done differently after thinking about it.

Write Your Scenario Here

Experienced Nurse Scenario

How Could it Be So Bad That a Mother Decides to Give up Her Children?

I was working as a school nurse in a really poor area of town. Welfare reform had been implemented for between 4 and 5 years. I had been making home visits to one family because the 10-year-old son was involved in a gang, had brought a knife to school, and threatened a teacher. After that, he was hospitalized in an inpatient mental health hospital for 3 days and released. Previously he had been in a detention facility for stealing car stereos. While he was there, he had a positive drug screen for marijuana and cocaine. He stayed away from home most nights. Unfortunately there weren't really any outpatient mental health services available in our community after the new county budget change.

This boy also had an 8-year-old brother who was a straight A student and was well liked by teachers and other children in the school. The two brothers fought a lot, but the younger one was a positive influence on the older one: When they were together, the 8-year old would say that he was going to call the police if the 10-year-old started doing something illegal. That usually stopped the 10-year-old for the time being. I had arranged to have the 10-year-old transferred to a continuation school for children, where he would have stricter limits on his behavior. The boys had an 11-month-old sister, and often the younger boy ended up taking care of her.

The entire family was Mien (a nationality in Southeast Asia like Vietnamese, Cambodian, Laotian) and the mother was deaf and mute, so I had to use sign language to communicate with her. She had been receiving state assistance for all the children. Just before the holiday season I went out to talk to her about how the 10-year-old was doing in his new school. She told me that the reimbursement she was receiving from the state for the boys just wasn't enough and she had decided to give both of them up. I asked her if anything else had happened recently that was upsetting her and she said no, but that the money just wasn't enough considering how much rent, food, and everything else in this area costs. There was no indication she was depressed, or any different than she had been on previous visits. I had always had the impression that she loved her sons and tried to the best of her ability to take care of them.

My first thought was that the 10-year old might be better off because a group home might be more successful in implementing a strict behavior control program which had been difficult for the mother. The next feeling I had was that the 8-year-old would feel really abandoned and his behavior could get worse. It didn't seem fair for him. He came into my office often just to say, "Hi," and I really liked him. I had a hard time understanding how a mother could just give her sons up because the level of reimbursement wasn't enough. I also felt bad for the mom because the older boy was a handful and very hard to manage. The mother told me she wanted the boys placed in an Asian group home and she wanted them to be together. I said I would come back and bring her telephone numbers if, after having time to think things over, that was what she really wanted. I also talked to her about temporary respite care so that she would have a chance to think things over and decide whether this was really what she wanted to do. I told her I would come back in 3 days. She said that in the meantime she wouldn't say anything to the boys.

When I got back to the school, I went in to talk to the psychologist because I was so upset about the mother's request. The psychologist said, "Well that's just typical. Some families have kids just to get money, and when the money might be cut, the kids don't matter. You need to let go of this and not let it get to you." That comment upset me even more, and I said I needed some alone time to think about the situation. I also mentioned that I was going to update the principal.

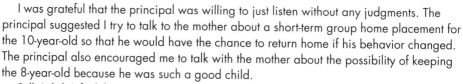

I was grateful that the principal was willing to just listen without any judgments. The principal suggested I try to talk to the mother about a short-term group home placement for the 10-year-old so that he would have the chance to return home if his behavior changed. The principal also encouraged me to talk with the mother about the possibility of keeping the 8-year-old because he was such a good child.

Still, I didn't feel that we came up with any real solutions for the mother. She would have a lot of difficulty going back to school or getting a job to support the boys, and her state support had been decreased. I had to think about how I was going to approach telling her that not all group homes were "outstanding," and that it might not be possible to keep the boys together, and it wasn't likely that an Asian group home could be found. I decided I would call my friends who also worked as school nurses to see if they could think of any options I had not considered. In the meantime I talked to the boy's teachers so that if something happened in class they would be alert to what the cause might be. What I told myself as I left work that day was that I know I had done everything possible to teach the mom ways to put limits on the 10-year-old's behavior, and I had been successful in getting him into a more structured school setting. I was determined not to give up advocating for the 8-year-old either.

THINKING IT THROUGH

1. What else did the school nurse need to know? What information was missing? (*Contextual awareness and deciding what to observe and consider*)

2. What emotional responses influenced how the school nurse was reacting in this situation? (*Contextual awareness and deciding what to observe and consider*)

3. What are other possible explanations for why the mother wanted to give the boys up? (*Exploring and imagining alternatives*)

4. Which possibility is most likely? Why are the others not as likely? (*Exploring and imagining alternatives*)

5. Were there other resources that needed to be mobilized? (*Exploring and imagining alternatives*)

6. What aspects of this situation required the most careful attention? (*Reflective skepticism/deciding what to do*)

7. In priority order, identify what you would have done in this situation and why. (*Reflective skepticism/deciding what to do*)

8. Contrast the attitudes and responses of the school nurse, the psychologist, and the principal. Which aspects of their behavior would you wish to incorporate or not incorporate into your own? (*Chapter reasoning problem*)

9. How would you have advocated for this mother? For the 8-year-old? For the 10-year-old? What sort of concerns would you have had for the baby and why? (*Chapter reasoning problem*)

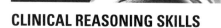

CLINICAL REASONING SKILLS

Comparing Beginners and Experienced Nurses

Think about the beginner scenarios, and then compare the experienced nurse's scenario related to the following:

- Emotional involvement with the patient

- Amount of detail recalled

- Assurance about the right thing to do

- Willingness to take action/effectiveness in advocating for the patients

- Continued concern about whether the correct action had been taken

List of Scenarios by Clinical Setting and by Beginner Reasoning Problem

Clinical Setting	Scenario Numbers
Medical-Surgical	2, 3, 4, 5, 7, 8, 9, 11
Maternal-Child	1, 6
Mental Health—School Nursing Scenario	10 and Experienced Nurse

Beginner Reasoning Problems	Scenario Numbers
Has a great sense of responsibility yet fears he/she could do harm	2, 4, 8, 10, 11
Does not persist in making things happen	1, 3, 4, 5, 7, 8, 10, 11
Unsure if the right things are getting done	2, 4, 6, 7, 10, 11
Feels others are not paying attention/are not engaged in the situation	1, 2, 3, 4, 5, 7, 8, 9, 10
Is not completely effective in advocating for the patient	1, 3, 4, 5, 6, 7, 8, 9, 10

Don't be hard on yourself. No one becomes a pro overnight.

tips!

REFERENCES

Adams, B.L. (1999). Nursing education for critical thinking: An integrative review. *Journal of Nursing Education, 38,* 111–119.

Beitz, J. (1998). Concept mapping: Navigating the learning process. *Nurse Educator, 23*(5), 35–41.

Benner, P., & Wrubel, J. (1989). *The Primacy of Caring.* Menlo Park, CA: Addison-Wesley.

Benner, P., Hooper-Kyriakidis, P., & Stannard, D. (1999). *Clinical Wisdom and Interventions in Critical Care: A Thinking-in-Action Approach.* Philadelphia: WB Saunders.

Benner, P., Tanner, C. & Chesla, C. (1996). *Experience in Nursing Practice: Caring, Clinical Judgement, and Ethics.* New York: Springer.

Brookfield, S. (1990). *The Skillful Teacher.* San Francisco, CA: Jossey Bass.

Cesarina, T., & Rebeschi, L. (1999). Critical thinking skills of baccalaureate nursing students at program entry and exit. *Nursing and Health Care Perspectives, 20*(30), 248–252.

Cob, P., & Bowers, J. (1999). Cognitive and situated learning perspectives in theory and practice. *Educational Researcher, 28*(2), 4–15.

Daley, B., Shaw, C., Balistrieri, T., Glasenapp, K., & Piacentine, L. (1999). Concept Maps: A strategy to teach and evaluate critical thinking. *Journal of Nursing Education 38*(1), 42–47.

Giarratano, G. (1997). Story as text for undergraduate curriculum. *Journal of Nursing Education, 36*(3), 128–134.

Gilligan, C. (1988). Remapping the moral domain: New images of self in relationship. In C. Gilligan, J. Victoria Ward, and J. McLean Taylor (Eds.), *Mapping the Moral Domain* (pp. 3–21). Cambridge: Harvard University Press.

Haffer, A., & Raingruber, B. (1998). Discovering confidence in clinical reasoning and critical thinking development in baccalaureate nursing students. *Journal of Nursing Education, 37*(2), 61–70.

Haffer, A. (1990). Beginning nurses' diagnostic reasoning behaviors derived from observation and verbal protocol analysis. *Dissertation Abstracts International, 52,* 160B, (University Microfilm No. 91–17, 892).

Kearney-Nunnery, R. (1997). *Advancing Your Career: Concepts of Professional Nursing.* Philadelphia: F.A. Davis.

Kirkpatrick, M.K., Ford, S., & Castelloe, B.P. (1997). Storytelling: An approach to client-centered care. *Nurse Educator, 22*(2), 38–40.

Magnussen, L., & Trotter, C. (1997). The reflective clinician. *Nurse Educator, 22*(3), 40–44.

Vetlesen, A. (1960). *Perception, Empathy and Judgment: An Inquiry into the Preconditions of Moral Performance.* Pennsylvania: The Pennsylvania State University Press.

INDEX

Page numbers followed by an f indicate figures.

A
Advocating for patient, 141–142, 171
Anticipation, 128

B
Brookfield, Stephen, critical thinking process(es)
    assumption recognition and analysis, 5–6
    contextual awareness, 4–6
    exploring and imaging alternatives, 4–6
    reflective skepticism/deciding what to do, 5–6

C
Clinical reasoning, 3, 14, 46, 53, 91, 136, 180
Community health scenario(s)
    freezing scenario, 36–39
    "staying open" scenario, 125–127
Critical thinking, definition of, 3
Critical thinking approach
    Brookfield's four critical thinking processes, 4–6
    journal, 8–9
    mind maps, 6–8, 7–8f

E
Ethical decision(s), 140–142
    in a nutshell, 171
    mind map for, 174–175
Ethical decision scenario(s)
    by beginner reasoning problem, 181
    Being Bounced Around, 164–166
    by clinical setting, 181
    Discharge Him, Suicidal or Not, 166–168
    Does the Order Always Come First?, 160–162
    How Could It Be So Bad That a Mother Decides to
        Give up Her Children?, 177–180
    I Can Still Hear Him Screaming, 141
    I Can't Believe He Said That!, 158–160

I Can't Believe She Hit Him, 153–155
I Wish I Had Let Her Family Stay, 148–150
Learning or Leering, 145–148
Neither My Patient Nor I Matter, 162–164
personal recollection of, 142–144, 175–176
The System Tied My Hands, 155–158
What to Do About Tom, 169–171
When Does the Patient Come First?, 150–153
Ethical dilemma, 145f
Experienced nurse scenario(s)
    How Could It Be So Bad That a Mother Decides to
        Give up Her Children?, 177–180
    I Just Knew Something Was Very Wrong, 90–92
    The Value of Staying Open, 133–137
    Where Do I Start? There's Always A New Crisis!, 51–53

F
Freezing, 12–13
    in a nutshell, 46
    mind map for, 16f, 47–49, 47–49f
Freezing scenario(s)
    by beginner reasoning problem, 54
    by clinical setting, 54
    A Float Day, 34–36
    Help! Here's Where I Get It, 39–45
    Help! I Can't Find My Clipboard, 20–22
    Help! I Can't Seem to Understand What He's Telling
        Me, 23–25
    Help! My Patient Can't Breathe! What's the Number
        for Respiratory?, 32–34
    I Forgot How to Give Oxygen!, 22–23
    I Thought I Was Prepared, 25–27
    I Wanted My Last Day to Be Good and I Feel Like I
        Failed, 27–30
    Passing Responsibility Can Be Positive, 30–32
    personal recollection of, 13–16, 49–50
    There's Something Wrong with the System, 36–39
    Where Do I Start? There's Always A New Crisis!, 51–53
    Why Didn't I Think to Ask That?, 17–19

J
Journal, reflective, 8–9

M

Maternal-child scenario(s)
  ethical decision scenarios, 145–148, 158–160
  freezing scenario, 20–23
  questioning scenarios, 72–74, 90–92
  "staying open" scenarios, 103–106, 118–120
Medical-surgical scenario(s)
  ethical decision scenarios, 148–158, 160–166, 169–171
  freezing scenarios, 17–19, 23–36
  questioning scenarios, 61–72, 74–83
  "staying open" scenarios, 100–103, 106–113, 116–120, 122–125, 133–137
Mental health scenario(s)
  ethical decision scenarios, 166–168, 177–180
  freezing scenario, 39–45
  questioning scenario, 72–74
  "staying open" scenarios, 114–115, 120–122
Mind map, 6–8, 7–8f
  for ethical decisions, 174–175
  for freezing, 16f, 47–49, 47–49f
  for questioning, 86–88, 86–87f
  for "staying open," 130–131

P

Picture mind map, 7, 7f
Previous experience, 97
Prioritizing, 128

Q

Questioning, 57, 60f
  in a nutshell, 83
  mind map for, 86–88, 86–87f
Questioning scenario(s)
  by beginner reasoning problem, 93
  by clinical setting, 93
  Do I Dare Ask for Help?, 57
  Do I Have the Right to Question This Order?, 78–81
  How Do I Give This Medication?, 76–78
  How Do You Even Begin to Ask Questions About Such Things?, 72–74
  I Just Knew Something Was Very Wrong, 90–92
  personal recollection of, 58–60, 88–89
  Shall I Implement This Standing Order?, 68–70
  She Might Get Back at Me If I Question Her, 74–76
  What Does He Mean, She Is Just 80?, 70–72
  What Does Waning In and Out Mean?, 61–62
  What Lab Work Do We Need?, 81–83
  Where's the PCA?, 63–65
  Why Wasn't I There for John?, 65–68

R

Reflective journal, 8–9
Routine, 12

S

School nursing scenario, ethical decision scenario, 177–180
"Staying open," 96–97, 100f
  in a nutshell, 128
  mind map for, 130–131
"Staying open" scenario(s)
  by beginner reasoning problem, 138
  by clinical setting, 138
  Don't Go with the First Thing That Comes to Mind, 97
  I Should Have Known, 123–125
  Learning to See What's Different, 110–113
  personal recollection of, 98–99, 131–132
  Seeing What Will Happen, 114–115
  Staying Open to Other Interpretations, 120–122
  Staying Open to the Patient's Feelings, 125–127
  Staying Open to What the Patient Wants, 108–110
  Stop That: Let Him Just Go for It, 103–106
  There's a Lot to Keep Track of, 106–108
  Thinking Backward to Figure Things Out, 100–103
  The Value of Staying Open, 133–137
  Was it Really an Air Bubble?, 118–120
  What Else Could Change in Just One Day?, 122–123
  What Else Should I Chart?, 116–118

U

Unexpected situation(s), 12, 13f

W

"What else . . ." question(s), 96–97
"What if . . ." question(s), 96–97, 128
Word mind map, 7, 8f

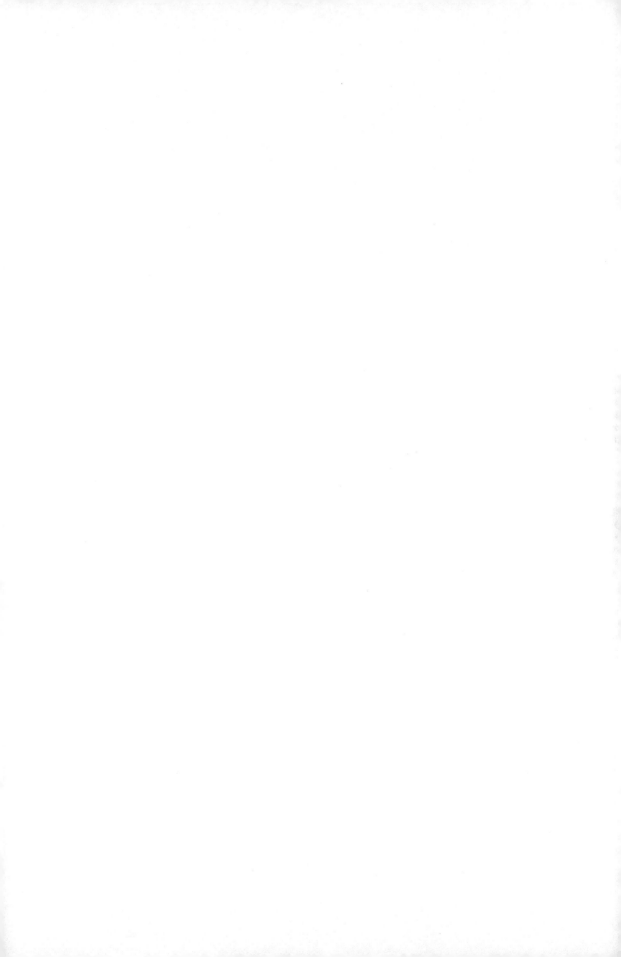